PHYSICIANS' GUIDE TO
THE Etiology & Treatment OF
DIARRHEA

Medical Economics Books
Oradell, New Jersey 07649

PHYSICIANS' GUIDE TO

THE Etiology & Treatment OF DIARRHEA

HORACIO JINICH, M.D., and TEODORO HERSH, M.D.

Edited by Harry Swartz, M.D.
Translated from the Spanish by Julia Baker, M.D.

Library of Congress Cataloging in Publication Data

Jinich, Horacio.
    Physicians' guide to etiology and treatment of
diarrhea.

      Translation of: Diarrea diagnostico y tratamiento.
      Includes index.
      1. Diarrhea.   I. Hersh, Teodoro.   II. Swartz,
Harry.   III. Title.   [DNLM: 1. Diarrhea—Etiology.
2. Diarrhea—Therapy.   WI 407 J61p]
RC862.D5J5613   616.3'427   81-18810
ISBN 0-87489-268-6   AACR2

Design by Penny Seldin

ISBN 0-87489-268-6

Medical Economics Company Inc.
Oradell, New Jersey 07649

Printed in the United States of America

Contents

Preface

The geographic ubiquity of diarrhea and its multiplicity of etiologies place it in the forefront of health problems around the world. It may vary in duration and intensity from a short-term nuisance to prolonged disability. It may presage a threat to life or may simply be an evanescent manifestation of momentary indiscretion.

Underlying diarrhea are a variety of pathologic processes of the gastrointestinal tract. In Part I of the book, the authors describe the tract's normal physiology and line out in direct and simple fashion the many deviations from normal that can result in diarrhea. Normal digestion, absorption, and metabolism of carbohydrates, fats, proteins, minerals, and fluids, as well as the gastrointestinal tract's motility, are described.

Having given the reader an overall conception of the mechanisms involved in diarrhea, the authors describe in Part II a practical approach to the patient with this symptom. They outline a classification of diarrhea based on anatomic, etiologic, and clinical data with special emphasis on the minutiae of history taking, so often overlooked in a busy office or clinic. They indicate the important characteristics of the stool to elicit, and tie these in with the gastrointestinal segment or extragastrointestinal organ or system responsible for diarrhea, including the patient's general health, eating habits, drug intake, past and family history, and emotional state. They point out what to look for in the physical, rectal, stool, and proctosigmoidoscopic examinations and what can be found by various laboratory tests, radiologic examination, and, when indicated, intestinal biopsy studies.

Part III summarizes clearly and simply the many clinical conditions in which diarrhea may be manifest, from dietary indiscretion to diabetes. Six appendices cover the practical details of proctosigmoidoscopy, peroral biopsy of the small intestine, duodenal aspiration, antidiarrheal medications, the components of a gluten-free diet, and total parenteral nutrition.

By integrating a large mass of information on an important but rarely studied topic, the authors have succeeded in their attempt to make diarrhea easily understandable in all its dimensions. The addition of concise summaries after most chapters is intended to highlight salient features of the text and, if desired, to serve as a basis for review. For all those who work in the health professions, this book will serve as a necessary aid and practical guide.

Harry Swartz, M.D.

Publisher's Notes

This book was originally published in 1977, under the title *Diarrea: Diagnóstico y Tratamiento,* by Francisco Mendez Otto Libreria Medicina, Mexico. The Spanish version was so well received that an English edition seemed highly desirable. The English version, however, is more than a translation. Dr. Jinich considerably updated and expanded the work for a North American medical audience before Dr. Baker translated it, with the editorial guidance of Dr. Swartz, into concise, idiomatic English. Dr. Swartz has also contributed chapter summaries that highlight salient features of the text and can serve as review material.

Horacio Jinich, M.D., is Professor of Medicine, Anahuac University School of Medicine, and head of the Department of Preventive Medicine and Diagnosis, American-British Cowdray Hospital, Mexico City. He also conducts a private practice specializing in diseases of the gastrointestinal tract. A fellow of both the American College of Physicians and the American College of Gastroenterologists, he was formerly Associate Professor of Medicine (Digestive Diseases), Emory University, Atlanta.

Teodoro Hersh, M.D., is Professor of Medicine (Digestive Diseases), Emory University, Atlanta.

Harry Swartz, M.D., served for 15 years as Clinical Professor of Medicine and Chief of the Allergy Clinic at the French and Polyclinic Medical School and Hospital in New York City. He is a prolific author on medical subjects and resides in Cuernavaca, Mexico.

Julia Baker, M.D., conducts a private practice specializing in allergy in Cuernavaca, Mexico.

PART I

NORMAL
AND PATHOLOGIC
PHYSIOLOGY

WATER AND ELECTROLYTE TRANSPORT IN THE INTESTINE

Normal physiology

1

The human intestine, both large and small, is a tube into whose lumen large amounts of water and electrolytes are delivered, and through whose walls important processes of transport and exchange with both vascular and extravascular systems take place. When the normal exchange process is disturbed, excessive amounts of water and electrolytes are lost and fecal matter becomes more liquid and is expelled more frequently, which results in diarrhea.

The amounts of water and electrolytes that normally reach the intestine each day are considerable, as can be seen in Table 1-1. It is clear, then, why the loss of these fluids should have an important effect on the hydroelectrolytic

TABLE 1-1

Approximate volumes of liquids and sodium that reach the intestinal lumen daily

Source	Liquids (liters)	Sodium (mmoles)
Food	2	50-150
Saliva	1	50
Gastric juice	2	100
Bile	1	200
Pancreatic juice	2	150

composition of the body tissues. Figures regarding liquids ingested, saliva, gastric juice, bile, and pancreatic juice are relatively easy to obtain and measure. There is controversy, however, regarding the amount of intestinal secretions. The exact amount is not known, but estimates of between 1 and 4 liters per day have been made. The source is thought to be the crypts of the intestinal epithelium. It is well known that absorption takes place in the villi.

Fortunately, the human intestine is a highly efficient system and is able to absorb more than 95 per cent of the liquids delivered into its lumen, transferring them to the extracellular spaces. Table 1-2 shows the relative proportions of liquids absorbed in the different segments of the intestine. Although the total amount of liquids absorbed successively by the jejunum, ileum, and colon decreases progressively, the rate of absorption—and thus its efficiency—increases from 50 per cent in the jejunum to more than 90 per cent in the colon.

The lumen of the jejunum is rich in nutrients: oligosaccharides, amino acids, oligopeptides, and fats in micellar suspension. The principal function of this segment of the intestine is to absorb these nutrients. Both water and electrolytes are absorbed along with the nutrients and are transported across the membrane. The nutrients are absorbed rapidly by either active transport or facilitated diffusion. The details of this process are still obscure. After water and electrolytes are absorbed in the jejunum, only a small part of

TABLE 1-2

Relative proportions of liquid absorbed in different segments of the intestine

Segment	Volume of liquid present (liters/day)	Volume of liquid absorbed (liters/day)	Proportion (%)
Jejunum	9	4-5	50
Ileum	4-5	3-4	75-80
Colon	1-2	0.9-1.8	> 90

what remains is transported actively by sodium pumps located in the membranes of epithelial cells.

Few nutrients reach the ileum. It's here, however, that water and electrolytes are mostly absorbed. The mechanisms are different than in the jejunum. The process in the ileum is active and is carried out by a neutral NaCl gradient in the brush border membrane. This process consists of a double exchange in which sodium is exchanged for hydrogen and chloride is exchanged for bicarbonate (Figure 1-1). In this way sodium and chloride are absorbed, while at the same time hydrogen and bicarbonate ions reach the intestine, forming carbonic acid. By means of the enzyme carbonic anhydrase, carbonic acid is broken down into carbon dioxide and water. These are readily absorbed.

The colon is the most efficient part of the intestine for absorption of water and sodium, one of its principal functions. Between 1 and 2 liters of intestinal fluids reach the colon daily. Since the feces contain only 100 to 200 ml of water, 90 to 99 per cent is absorbed here. Likewise, out of 200 mmoles of sodium that reach the colon, only 5 mmoles are excreted. The transport system is active and is under the influence of the adrenal steroids, especially aldosterone. It has been calculated that the colon can absorb a maximum of 2.4 liters of water, 400 mmoles of sodium, and 560 mmoles of chloride daily. For diarrhea to occur, volumes of water and electrolytes in excess of these figures must reach the normally functioning colon.

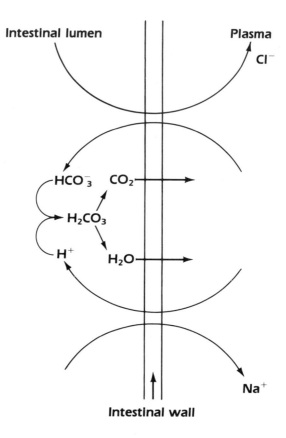

FIGURE 1-1 **Active transport of electrolytes in and out of the ileum**

Potassium is passively absorbed in the small intestine and, in small amounts, in the colon. This ion may be secreted in the colon as a component of intestinal mucus. The daily fecal excretion of potassium is 6 to 12 mmoles, and that of sodium, 2 to 5 mmoles.

Bicarbonate is secreted by the ileum during the chloride-bicarbonate exchange. Some of it reacts with hydrogen in the intestinal lumen, with the formation of CO_2 and water, and some reaches the large intestine, where it combines with organic acids produced by bacterial fermentation of the carbohydrates that have not been absorbed in the small intestine.

The stomach plays an important role in the regulation of electrolyte transport during digestion. Digestive juices are isotonic and consequently do not disturb the osmotic equilibrium that exists between the intestinal lumen and extracellular spaces. On the other hand, many foods and beverages are not isotonic. Some, such as water, are hypotonic. Some are hypertonic; their presence in the jejunum pulls in large amounts of water from the extracellular spaces. One of the stomach's most important functions is to prevent this from happening: Its walls are impermeable to water and electrolytes and its emptying rate is under the control of osmoreceptors located in the duodenum.

Bibliography

Edmonds CJ, Pilcher D: Sodium transport mechanisms of the large intestine. In *Transport Across the Intestine* (Borland WL, Samuel PD, eds), pp. 43–57. Edinburgh: Churchill Livingstone, 1972

Hendrix TR, Bayless TM: Digestion: Intestinal secretion. *Annu Rev Physiol* 32:139, 1970

Krejs GJ, Fordtran JS: Physiology and pathophysiology of ion and water movement in the human intestine. In *Gastrointestinal Disease* (Sleisenger MH, Fordtran JS, eds), 2nd ed, vol 1, pp 297–313. Philadelphia: Saunders, 1978

Phillips SF: Diarrhea: A current view of the pathophysiology. *Gastroenterology* 63:495, 1972

Phillips SF: Diarrhea: Pathogenesis and diagnostic techniques. *Postgrad Med* 57:65, 1975

Phillips SF, Giller J: The contribution of the colon to electrolyte and water conservation in man. *J Lab Clin Med* 81:733, 1976

Schedl HP: Water and electrolyte transport. Clinical aspects. *Med Clin North Am* 58:1429, 1974

Sweadner KJ, Golden SM: Active transport of sodium and potassium ions. *N Engl J Med* 302:777, 1980

Turnberg LA: Electrolyte absorption from the colon. *Gut* 11:1049, 1970

Turnberg LA, Breberdorf FA, Morawski SS, et al: Interrelationship of chloride, bicarbonate, sodium and hydrogen transport in the human ileum. *J Clin Invest* 49:557, 1970

SUMMARY

Diarrhea results when there is an interference with the transport of water and electrolytes through the intestinal wall, causing increased liquidity and expulsion of feces.

Eight liters of liquid derived from food, saliva, gastric juice, bile, and pancreatic juice, and 1 to 4 liters from intestinal secretions representing 550 to 650 mmoles of sodium, reach the intestine daily. Of this amount, 95 per cent is absorbed, there being a downward gradient from the jejunum to the colon. In contrast, the percentage absorption follows an upward gradient.

The jejunum is rich in nutrients, which are absorbed with water and electrolytes by active transport or facilitated diffusion. A very small part of the remnant is transported actively by sodium pumps in the epithelial membrane.

The ileum contains few nutrients. Here, water and electrolytes are largely absorbed actively via a neutral sodium chloride carrier in the brush-border membrane. Sodium is exchanged with hydrogen, and chloride with bicarbonate. Thus sodium and chloride are absorbed and hydrogen and bicarbonate form carbonic acid, which is broken down by carbonic anhydrase to water and carbon dioxide, also readily absorbed.

The largest percentage of water and sodium is absorbed by the colon. It is estimated that the colon can absorb 2.4 liters of water, 400 mmoles of sodium, and 560 mmoles of chloride daily. More than these amounts in a normal colon result in diarrhea.

Potassium is passively absorbed in the intestine, its daily fecal excretion being 6 to 12 mmoles, while that of sodium is 2 to 5 mmoles.

The stomach juices are isotonic, its walls impermeable to water and electrolytes. Its emptying rate is controlled by osmoreceptors in the duodenum. It maintains the tonicity of its contents, and therefore the proper direction of absorption from the gastrointestinal tract.

Pathophysiology of water and electrolyte transport

2

Diarrhea, the abnormally frequent expulsion of feces of decreased consistency, is due to disturbances in the transport of water and electrolytes in the intestine. At least four major mechanisms have been proven:

1. Increased luminal osmolarity: osmotic diarrhea
2. Increased electrolyte secretion: secretory diarrhea
3. Decreased electrolyte absorption
4. Deranged intestinal motility (i.e., decreased transit time).

Several other possible mechanisms lack definitive proof: changes in mucosal morphology, increases in mucosal permeability, and changes in mesenteric blood flow.

It's important to emphasize that in most specific diarrheal diseases more than one mechanism may be responsible for the production of diarrhea.

Osmotic diarrhea

Osmotic diarrhea is caused by accumulation of solutes that produce a hypertonic solution in the intestinal lumen. These may be:

1. Foreign, poorly absorbable solutes such as saline laxatives
2. Foods of high osmotic pressure that cannot be absorbed because of lack of enzymes to break them down
3. Inhibition of intestinal absorption of a dietary nonelectrolyte.

Table 2-1 lists the causes of osmotic diarrhea. Whatever the cause, the presence of unabsorbed solutes of relative small molecular size causes a net displacement of water from the plasma into the intestinal lumen.

Dietary indiscretion
Eating a large beefsteak does not usually cause digestive problems in a person who is healthy. But if he consumes three or four glasses of milk and half a dozen doughnuts, or eats a large amount of unripe fruit, he's likely to pay for his voracity with a disagreeable though transitory diarrhea. While the meat reaches the duodenum in normal or hypotonic concentration, the other combinations of foods are frankly hypertonic because of their high content of disaccharide molecules.

Rapid gastric emptying
As stated in the previous chapter, one of the stomach's most important functions is to prevent hypertonic food solutions from reaching the intestines. This is accomplished by duodenal osmoreceptors that regulate the stomach's emptying. When part or all of the stomach has been removed or a pyloroplasty or gastroenterostomy has been performed, this mechanism is interfered with and diarrhea results. The

TABLE 2-1

Causes of osmotic diarrhea

1. Dietary indiscretion
2. Rapid gastric emptying
3. Deficient intestinal absorption
4. Enzyme deficiencies
5. Osmotic laxatives

rapid passage of hypertonic food solutions into the jejunum pulls in large amounts of water and electrolytes from the extracellular spaces. Diarrhea, intestinal distention, and hypovolemia are the results of rapid emptying of the stomach.

Deficient intestinal absorption
Many pathologic processes of the human small intestine give rise to the malabsorption syndrome, both primary and secondary, which will be explained in Chapter 22. In this condition the intestinal lumen is filled with molecules that cannot be absorbed. These include molecules resulting from the enzymatic action of pancreatic juice and the intestinal epithelial cells: mono- and oligosaccharides, amino acids, oligopeptides, and fats in micellar suspension. Minerals, vitamins, and water are also present. Many of these nutrients, especially mono- and oligosaccharides, cause osmotic diarrhea.

Enzyme deficiencies
One of the most important causes of osmotic diarrhea is lactase deficiency. Lactase is the intestinal enzyme necessary to break down the disaccharide lactose into the monosaccharides glucose and galactose. Lactase is synthesized in the cells of the fetal intestinal epithelium from the third month on, and reaches its maximum production at birth and during infancy. Some human ethnic groups, especially Europeans and their descendants, maintain high levels of lactase activity during all their adult lives. Other groups suffer a

gradual decrease in the activity of this enzyme, which may reach its lowest level during either childhood, adolescence, or adult life. This deficiency results in osmotic diarrhea whenever milk or other foods rich in lactose exceed the enzymatic capacity of the intestines. Lactose in solution in the small intestine is hypertonic and behaves as an osmotic laxative (see below), inducing net fluid accumulation. Ethnic groups deficient in lactase include Jews, American Indians, and blacks.

Much less frequently found than lactase deficiency in adults is alactasia in children due to a total or partial congenital deficiency. The clinical picture consists of diarrhea that responds only to omitting all milk, both maternal milk and cow's milk. A deficiency of lactase and other disaccharidases may be present in many diseases associated with malabsorption. An acquired, though usually transitory, deficiency of these enzymes may occur in intestinal infections and infestations with parasites such as acute bacterial and viral gastroenteritis or giardiasis.

Rare cases of sucrase deficiency alone, and of combined sucrase and isomaltase deficiencies, have been described. Cases of congenital inability to absorb glucose and galactose have been reported. In all these the pathophysiology is the same: osmotic diarrhea.

Osmotic laxatives
Saline laxatives such as sodium or magnesium sulfate, various alkaline medications containing magnesium salts, and unabsorbed polyhydrolate compounds such as sorbitol and lactulose produce catharsis by osmotic action, drawing large amounts of water from the extracellular space into the jejunal lumen.

Clinical characteristics of osmotic diarrhea
Osmotic diarrhea has certain clinical and biochemical characteristics:

1. The ileum and colon retain the ability to absorb sodium, since their pores are smaller than those of the jejunum and since this ion is absorbed by an active process. Thus the concentration of sodium in the stool is

less than in the plasma, and since water is lost in excess of sodium, there is a tendency to hypernatremia.

2. The stool contains more potassium than sodium, since the colon conserves sodium but not potassium.

3. The osmolarity of the stool is due to electrolytes and nonelectrolytes such as oligosaccharides. Consequently, the electrolyte concentration of the stool is less than its osmolarity. Electrolyte concentration can be calculated by adding the milliequivalents of sodium plus potassium (cations) to chloride and bicarbonate (anions). It's better, however, to measure only the concentration of cations and multiply it by 2, since part of the bicarbonate has combined with organic radicals.

4. Unabsorbed oligosaccharides are fermented by bacteria in the colon, making the feces acid. This is easily proved by measuring their pH.

5. Diarrhea stops if the patient stops eating. A fast of 24 to 72 hours, giving only intravenous fluids, will accomplish this.

Secretory diarrhea

Secretory diarrhea may be produced, at least on theoretical grounds, by either passive or active increased electrolyte secretion. Passive secretion is caused by increased hydrostatic and tissue pressure. It may explain the diarrhea seen in cases of extracellular volume expansion, elevation of mesenteric venous pressure, lymphatic obstruction, mucosal inflammation, and intestinal ischemia. Active electrolyte secretion is the most important cause of secretory diarrhea. Theoretically this might result from a decrease in the movement of ions and water from the lumen to the plasma, or from an increase in their movement from the plasma to the lumen. Causes of secretory diarrhea are listed in Table 2-2.

Diarrhea from excessive secretion may have its origin in the stomach, small intestine, or colon.

Secretory diarrhea of gastric origin occurs in some cases of gastrinoma, or Zollinger-Ellison syndrome. The enormous amounts of gastric juice produced as a result of stimulation by gastrin cause diarrhea, probably by a number of mechanisms: The volume of gastric secretion is increased;

TABLE 2-2

Causes of secretory diarrhea

1. Infectious
   a. Toxigenic: *Vibrio cholerae,* some *Escherichia coli, Shigella dysenteriae* I, *Staphylococcus aureus, Clostridium perfringens, Pseudomonas aeruginosa*
   b. Invasive: *Shigella* spp, *Salmonella* spp, *E. coli, Entamoeba histolytica*

2. Neoplastic
   a. Villous adenoma
   b. Ganglioneuroma
   c. Medullary carcinoma of the thyroid
   d. Gastrinoma (Zollinger-Ellison syndrome)
   e. Syndrome of watery diarrhea, hypokalemia, and hypochlorhydria (pancreatic cholera)
   f. Carcinoid syndrome

3. Cathartics

the pH of the small intestine is decreased sufficiently to affect mucosal structure and function; digestion of fat is impaired by the abnormally low pH in the jejunum, leading to steatorrhea. Hypergastrinemia may be due to direct humoral stimulus of secretion in the small intestine.

Infectious causes of secretory diarrhea

Bacterial pathogens are responsible for the great majority of acute diarrheal illnesses. They may be divided into two distinct groups: the noninvasive, toxigenic microorganisms, which cause no detectable mucosal damage, and the invasive pathogens, which penetrate and damage the gut mucosa. These last pathogens have relatively little effect on small-bowel fluid transport; whatever diarrhea they produce is probably secondary to passive secretion. The noninvasive bacteria produce toxins that cause the small intestine to produce fluids in amounts that overwhelm the absorptive capacity of the colon, resulting in diarrhea.

Cholera is the prototype of the toxigenic diarrheas. The cholera enterotoxin is a complex protein of 84,000 mol wt, composed of a binding and an activating moiety. The binding moiety binds to the epithelial cell wall and, after a lag period of 15 to 30 minutes, the activating moiety stimulates adenylate cyclase by a nicotinamide adenine dinucleotide (NAD)-dependent mechanism. The resultant increased intracellular cyclic adenosine monophosphate (cyclic AMP) is responsible for secretion of isotonic fluid by the entire length of the small bowel. Besides stimulating active anion secretion, cyclic AMP affects intestinal ion transport by inhibiting the brush-border carrier, which is responsible for neutral NaCl influx across the brush border of the intestine. In this way, cyclic AMP alters both absorptive and secretory processes while it inhibits the influx of NaCl into villous epithelial cells. It stimulates active Cl^- secretion in epithelial cells of the crypts. Recent studies provide excellent support for the hypothesis that cyclic AMP may affect intestinal ion transport by altering intracellular calcium pools and thus increasing mucosal chloride permeability.

The specific brush-border carrier for sodium chloride, a nucleotide, is inhibited by increased concentrations of cyclic AMP. However, it does not diminish the capacity of the cell's sodium pump, so that if an alternative pathway for sodium entry across the brush border could be used, salt and water absorption would be restored. Glucose does not interfere with the specific effects of cyclic AMP on active ion transport, but independently stimulates salt and water absorption.

E. coli may produce either a heat-labile or a heat-stable toxin, or both. As with cholera, ingested *E. coli* proliferate in the upper portion of the small bowel, and the pathophysiologic effects are due primarily to the action of the enterotoxins on the epithelial cells of the small bowel. The heat-labile toxin is structurally similar to cholera enterotoxin and displays similar kinetics of activation of adenylate cyclase and fluid secretion. The *E. coli* heat-stable toxin appears to act via stimulation of guanylate cyclase.

The other two major enterotoxin-induced diarrheal diseases are pathophysiologically different from cholera and *E. coli* gastroenteritis. The mechanism by which staphylococcal enterotoxin causes gut fluid loss has not been clearly delineated. It appears to be mediated, at least in part, by hyperperistalsis caused by action of absorbed enterotoxin on the autonomic nervous system. The *Cl. perfringens* enterotoxin causes secretion of isotonic fluid into the small bowel by a mechanism, as yet unexplained, which involves neither adenylate cyclase nor guanylate cyclase.

Neoplastic causes of secretory diarrhea

Vasoactive intestinal peptide (VIP), the polypeptide responsible for many (but not all) cases of the watery diarrhea, hypokalemia, and hypochlorhydria syndrome (pancreatic cholera), stimulates adenylate cyclase and increases mucosal cyclic AMP. Thus, it stimulates net Cl^- secretion and inhibits NaCl absorption.

Some tumors, such as medullary carcinoma of the thyroid, secrete prostaglandins (PG, PGE in particular) that affect fluid and electrolyte transport and increase mucosal cyclic AMP in a manner similar to VIP and cholera enterotoxin. In contrast, calcitonin, serotonin, gastric inhibitory peptide, and cholecystokinin affect the secretory process through other, as yet unidentified, mechanisms.

Villous adenomas, when they occur in the distal part of the colon, cause diarrhea by secreting sodium, potassium, and water. Sometimes this secretion is so abundant that patients suffer from hypokalemia and dehydration.

Laxatives such as the dihydroxy bile acids (deoxycholic acid and chenodeoxycholic acid) and hydroxy fatty acids (ricinoleic acid, the active ingredient of castor oil) have several effects on intestinal function: increasing mucosal cyclic AMP levels, stimulating active Cl^- secretion, increasing mucosal permeability, affecting myoelectric activity, and altering the mucosal structure.

Clinical characteristics of secretory diarrhea

Several characteristics differentiate secretory diarrheas from osmotic diarrheas:

1. Large volume of diarrheal stools
2. Electrolytic concentration only slightly less than osmolarity, since osmolarity in diarrheal stools is almost entirely due to secreted ions

3. Neutral fecal pH, as there are no fermentation products
4. Sodium losses greater than potassium losses
5. Failure to stop with fasting.

Decreased electrolyte absorption

Diarrhea caused by decreased electrolyte absorption is seen in patients with sprue, either celiac or tropical. In either kind of sprue, there's a marked decrease in absorptive area from villous atrophy, in addition to a definite decrease in the diameter of the pores of the jejunum. Other factors contributing to the diarrhea of celiac sprue include both secondary lactase deficiency, which is related to the histologic abnormalities of the brush border, and steatorrhea.

Congenital chloridorrhea is caused by a defect in the active interchange of chloride and bicarbonate that normally takes place in the ileum and colon. Sodium-hydrogen exchange, however, does take place. The results are fecal loss of excessive amounts of chloride in the diarrheal stools, exceeding the combined loss of sodium and potassium; acidification of the intestinal contents, which is not neutralized by bicarbonate; and systemic alkalosis.

Bile salts, when they are able to function normally in the enterohepatic cycle, do not give rise to diarrhea. When deconjugated and dehydroxylated, however, bile salts inhibit the absorption of water and electrolytes. This happens when there is overgrowth of intestinal bacteria that alter the bile salts, or when bile salts, which should have been absorbed in the terminal ileum, reach the colon instead. Diarrhea in these cases is caused by inhibition of the normal active absorption of ions.

Hydroxylated fatty acids also inhibit active absorption of ions in the intestine. Ricinoleic acid, the active principle of castor oil, is a hydroxylated fatty acid, which explains its cathartic effect. When fatty acids are poorly absorbed, bacteria may convert them to hydroxylated fatty acids. This would explain the diarrhea that accompanies steatorrhea in many of these cases. Table 2-3 summarizes the relationships between electrolyte and fluid balance in osmotic and secretory diarrhea.

TABLE 2-3

Fecal electrolytes and their effects on water and electrolyte balance in osmotic and secretory diarrhea

Secretory diarrhea	Osmotic diarrhea
Composition of stools	
Na > K	K > Na
2 (Na + K) ~ mOsm	2 (Na + K) < mOsm
pH ~ 7	pH ~ 5
Water and electrolyte balance	
Dehydration	Dehydration
Hyponatremia	Hypokalemia

Deranged intestinal motility

Changes of intestinal motor activity have long been considered a frequent cause of diarrhea. However, most investigators are now unwilling to assign a primary role to changes of intestinal motility in the genesis of increased stool water excretion. Although a decrease in intestinal transit time may decrease electrolyte absorption, it's doubtful that net fluid and electrolyte accumulation could ever result from an increase in motor activity. However, the increase in intestinal volume secondary to net fluid accumulation may be responsible for some of the motor abnormalities observed in certain diarrheal diseases.

Diarrhea in the carcinoid syndrome used to be considered an example of a primary motility disorder induced by serotonin stimulation. It has been demonstrated that this humoral agent in fact induces net fluid and electrolyte accumulation.

Opiates, whose effectiveness as antidiarrheal agents was believed to be secondary to their action on smooth muscles, may be therapeutic through a different mechanism. It has been demonstrated that the endogenous opioid peptide met-enkephalin stimulates active Na^+ and Cl^- absorption.

That the importance of deranged motility in the etiology of diarrhea has not been definitely settled is exemplified by the diarrhea of irritable bowel syndrome and hyperthyroidism, for which no other explanation has been offered. Also, it's likely that hyperperistalsis may account for the diarrhea caused by staphylococcal enterotoxin.

It should be stressed again that the majority of diarrheas are not of just one type, but rather are a combination of the various mechanisms described here. There still remain many obscure and controversial areas in this important field of normal and pathologic physiology.

Bibliography

Binder HJ: Net fluid and electrolyte secretion: The pathophysiologic basis for diarrhea. In *Mechanisms of Intestinal Secretion* (Binder HJ, ed), p 1. New York: Liss, 1979

Binder HJ: Pharmacology of laxatives. *Annu Rev Pharmacol Toxicol* 17:355, 1977

Carpenter CCJ: Mechanisms of bacterial diarrhea. *Am J Med* 68:313, 1980

Field M: Intestinal secretion. *Gastroenterology* 66:1063, 1974

Fordtran JS: Speculations on the pathogenesis of diarrhea. *Fed Proc* 26: 1405, 1967

Kregs GJ, Fordtran JS: Diarrhea. In *Gastrointestinal Disease* (Sleisenger MH, Fordtran JS, eds), 2nd ed, vol 1, pp 313–335. Philadelphia: Saunders, 1978

Phillips SF: Diarrhea: A current view of the pathophysiology. *Gastroenterology* 63:495, 1972

Phillips SF: Diarrhea: Pathogenesis and diagnostic techniques. *Postgrad Med* 57:65, 1975

SUMMARY

Diarrhea has four major pathophysiologic mechanisms:

1. Increased luminal osmolarity causes osmotic diarrhea. This can be produced by accumulation of hypertonic solutes in the intestine, the result of dietary indiscretion, rapid gastric emptying, deficient intestinal ab-

sorption, enzyme deficiency (congenital lactase deficiency is one of the most important in this category), or
osmotic laxatives.

2. Secretory diarrhea may originate in the stomach,
   small intestine, or colon as a result of toxic or invasive
   microorganisms, neoplasms, or cathartics, causing
   passive or active increased electrolyte secretion. Bacterial pathogens are responsible for the greater majority
   of acute diarrheas, *V. cholerae* being the prototype organism of the toxic, noninvasive diarrheas. *E. coli* acts
   in a similar fashion. *Staphylococcus* and *Clostridium,*
   although differing from the preceding two in their
   mode of action, belong to this category. Neoplasms, as
   villous adenomas, ganglioneuromas, medullary carcinoma of the thyroid, gastrinomas, carcinoids, "pancreatic cholera," and cathartics (dihydroxy bile acids and
   castor oil) also produce this category of diarrhea.

3. Decreased electrolyte absorption is seen in celiac and
   tropical sprue and in congenital chloridorrhea due to
   anatomical or biochemical interference with electrolyte balance. Hydroxylated bile salts and castor oil may
   belong to this category also.

4. Changes of intestinal motor activity are thought by
   some to be due to a decrease in intestinal transit time,
   although this is probably not the cause. The pathogenesis of diarrhea due to irritable colon and hyperthyroidism, put in this category, is still unknown.

Hydroelectrolytic effects of diarrhea

3

It is not difficult to predict the effect of diarrhea on water and electrolyte balance. The loss of water results in dehydration. Dehydration is isotonic if the loss of electrolytes is in proportion to water loss, hypotonic if the patient receives water or hypotonic solutions by mouth or intravenously (or if there is excessive secretion of antidiuretic hormone), or hypertonic in cases of osmotic diarrhea, in which the patient loses more water than he does electrolytes.

Hypokalemia can occur in acute diarrhea, especially of osmotic origin. It also occurs in chronic diarrhea when the colon is able to absorb sodium but not potassium. This is more severe in cases of secondary hyperaldosteronism. Isolated potassium depletion is frequently found in people who practice chronic laxative abuse.

The acid-base balance in diarrhea may shift from acidosis to alkalosis, depending on the loss of bicarbonate or acids, as well as on the secondary effects of hypokalemia, fasting ketosis, shock, and renal failure.

Bibliography

Gamble JL: *Chemical Anatomy, Physiology and Pathology of Extracellular Fluid.* Cambridge, Mass: Harvard University Press, 1949

Schwartz WB, Relman AS: Metabolic and renal studies in chronic potassium depletion resulting from overuse of laxatives. *J Clin Invest* 32:258, 1953

CARBOHYDRATE DIGESTION

Normal physiology

4

The carbohydrates in the human diet are starch, glycogen, cellulose, sucrose, and lactose. Starch is a mixture of two glucose polymers, amylose and amylopectin. Amylose is a linear chain of glucose molecules in which the first carbon of one molecule is linked to the fourth carbon of the next molecule, and so on successively (1,4 bonds). Amylopectin is also made up of a chain of glucose molecules with 1,4 linkages but in addition it has lateral chains with 1,6 linkages.

In animal foods, glycogen takes the place of starch in plant foods. Its structure is very similar to amylopectin's. Glycogen has little nutritional value because most of it is catabolized when the animal is slaughtered.

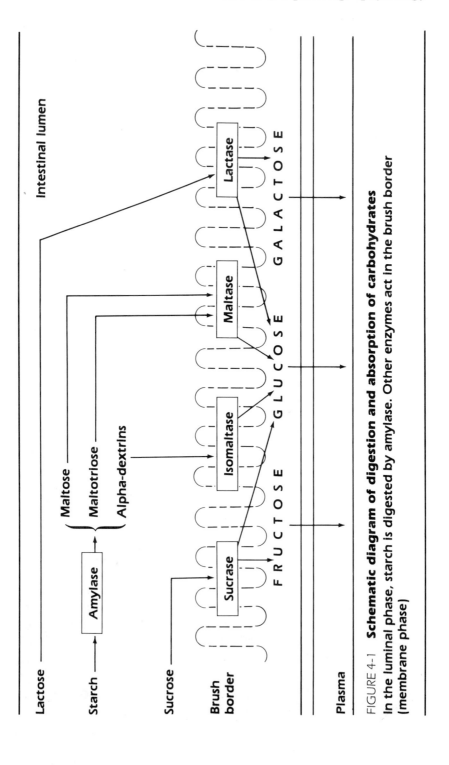

FIGURE 4-1 **Schematic diagram of digestion and absorption of carbohydrates**
In the luminal phase, starch is digested by amylase. Other enzymes act in the brush border (membrane phase)

Cellulose is the most abundant polysaccharide in the vegetable kingdom. Unlike starch, it is made up of molecules of monosaccharides that, being of the beta type, are not acted upon by human digestive enzymes.

Sucrose and lactose are disaccharides. Sucrose is ordinary sugar and consists of a molecule of glucose and a molecule of fructose. Lactose, or milk sugar, is found in milk and many of its derivatives and is made up of a molecule of glucose and another of galactose.

Digestion of carbohydrates occurs in two places: in the lumen of the gut (intraluminal phase) and in the membrane of the intestinal epithelium (membrane phase). Figure 4-1 is a schematic diagram of the phases of carbohydrate digestion.

Intraluminal digestion consists essentially of incomplete hydrolysis of starch and glycogen by means of the pancreatic enzyme amylase. This endo-enzyme attacks the 1,4 bonds, but not the 1,6 bonds, of amylose and amylopectin, thus liberating the disaccharide maltose, which is made up of two molecules of glucose; the trisaccharide maltotriose; and a set of branched oligosaccharides called alpha-dextrins. These alpha-dextrins are the result of the inability of amylase to attack 1,6 bonds, the starting point of the amylopectin branches. Theoretically, salivary ptyalin (amylase) should participate in the digestion of starch. This is not the case, however, since amylase actually is inactivated by gastric juice.

When the intraluminal stage of carbohydrate digestion is completed, the lumen of the gut contains molecules of maltose, maltotriose, and alpha-dextrins, as well as molecules of sucrose and lactose. These are acted upon in the small intestine by enzymes, disaccharidases, present in the epithelium of the villi. Maltose and maltotriose are broken down by various enzymes, called maltases, into glucose. The alpha-dextrins are acted upon by isomaltase; sucrose, by sucrase or invertase; and lactose, by lactase.

The monosaccharides resulting from the membrane stage of digestion of carbohydrates are glucose, galactose, and fructose. They are absorbed efficiently in the jejunum, and to a lesser extent in the ileum, by means of the epithelial cells of the intestinal villi. Glucose and galactose are actively transported by "carriers" that are not yet identified but are probably made up of proteins of the same cellular membrane. This active transport of monosaccharides is linked in some way with the simultaneous transport of sodium and water. Fructose is also rapidly absorbed by means of facilitated diffusion, a mechanism independent of the transport of glucose and galactose.

Bibliography

Crane RG: Absorption of sugars. In *Handbook of Physiology* (Code CF, ed), vol 3, p. 1323. Washington, DC: American Physiological Society, 19 69

Gray GM: Carbohydrate digestion and absorption: Role of the small intestine. *N Engl J Med* 292:1225, 1975

SUMMARY

Carbohydrate digestion takes place in the lumen of the intestine and in the membrane of its epithelium. Within the gut, starch and glycogen are incompletely hydrolyzed by pancreatic amylase, liberating maltose, maltotriose, and alpha-dextrins. In addition, dietary sucrose and lactose are present in the gut. Disaccharidases of the epithelial villi break down the maltose and maltotriose into glucose. Alpha-dextrins are acted upon by isomaltase, sucrose by sucrase or invertase, and lactose by lactase. The resulting monosaccharides are glucose, galactose, and fructose. Absorption occurs in the jejunum and ileum, more effectively in the former.

Pathophysiology of digestion and absorption of carbohydrates

5

Both monosaccharides, resulting from the membrane stage of carbohydrate digestion, and disaccharides, which precede them in the digestive process, are molecules with great osmotic power. If not rapidly absorbed, they can interfere with the normal exchange of fluids and electrolytes in the intestine. What would happen if 300 gm of carbohydrates of a normal diet underwent normal intraluminal digestion but no membrane digestion? Two hundred grams of starch would yield 382 mOsmoles of disaccharides, while 100 gm of sucrose and lactose would yield another 280 mOsmoles, making a total of 662 mOsmoles. Without disaccharidase activity, this mass of disaccharide molecules would pull 4.8 liters of liquid into the

TABLE 5-1

Defects of digestion and absorption of carbohydrates

---

1. Defects in the intraluminal phase (amylase deficiency)
   Transitory deficiency of amylase in the newborn
   Obstruction of the pancreatic duct

2. Defects in the membrane phase
   Lactase deficiency
      Acquired
      Congenital
      Secondary to epithelial damage
   Deficiency of all disaccharidases (secondary
      to epithelial damage)
   Deficiency of sucrase and isomaltase
   Deficiency of trehalase

3. Deficiencies of absorption of glucose and galactose
   Congenital
   Acquired

---

intestine. On the other hand, if disaccharidase action were normal but the monosaccharides could not be absorbed, the results would be even worse, since 300 gm of carbohydrate correspond to 1,700 mOsmoles of monosaccharides. The clinical result of these severe enzymatic deficiencies would be osmotic diarrhea. The arrival of carbohydrates in the colon would, in turn, produce a chain of pathophysiologic changes: bacterial fermentation of carbohydrates, production of lactic acid, other short-chain fatty acids, and hydrogen gas, followed by the osmotic effect of the fatty acids, and lowering of the pH. Table 5-1 summarizes defects in absorption and digestion of carbohydrates.

Amylase deficiencies are exceedingly rare. They occur transiently in newborns, but are seen in adults only if there is total obstruction of the pancreatic duct. In destructive lesions of the pancreas, no matter how advanced they may be, enough pancreatic enzyme is produced to take care of digestive needs. This ability of the pancreas always to secrete enough amylase is remarkable. Lactase deficiency, however, is a frequent problem. It can be stated without exaggeration that a large portion of the world's adult population has the acquired form of this deficiency. Congenital forms exist in infants. This is discussed in detail in Chapter 39.

Any disease that diffusely damages the mucous membrane of the small intestine may cause transient deficiencies in the disaccharidases. These enzymes may disappear and then reappear when the primary disease subsides. This happens in celiac sprue, tropical sprue, giardiasis, acute viral gastroenteritis, and mucosal damage from drugs such as neomycin and para-aminosalicylic acid. Of all the disaccharidases, lactase is the most readily affected and the last to reappear. Deficiency of sucrase and isomaltase occurs in a congenital disease, with onset in infancy developing as soon as the first foods containing sucrose and isomaltose are ingested. Trehalose is a disaccharide found in fresh mushrooms. Its ingestion by individuals with a deficiency of the enzyme trehalase produces diarrhea. Intolerance to maltose fortunately does not occur, probably because various enzymes have maltase activity.

Deficient absorption of glucose and galactose may be hereditary and congenital, in which case it is extremely dangerous, threatening the life of the infant. On the other hand, it may be acquired and transitory, as a result of infectious gastroenteritis. Treatment consists of eliminating all carbohydrates, with the exception of fructose.

Bibliography

Gray IM: Intestinal digestion and maldigestion of dietary carbohydrates. *Annu Rev Med* 22:391, 1971

Marks JF, Norton JB, Fordtran JS: Glucose-galactose malabsorption. *J Pediatr* 69:225, 1966

Olsen WA: Carbohydrate absorption. *Med Clin North Am* 58:1387, 1974

SUMMARY

The disaccharides and monosaccharides are molecules of great osmotic power. If not rapidly absorbed, they would pull great quantities of fluid into the intestinal lumen, resulting in a severe osmotic diarrhea. In addition, carbohydrates in the colon would result in fermentation, the formation of lactic acid, short-chain fatty acids, and hydrogen gas, and lowering of the pH. Proper digestion and absorption of carbohydrates may be deranged by any of several deficiencies. Amylase deficiency (intraluminal) is rare. More common are membrane-phase defects: lactase deficiency, which is very common in adults; disaccharidase deficiency due to any disease damaging the intestinal mucosa; sucrase and isomaltase deficiency, with onset in infancy; and deficiency of trehalase, an enzyme that breaks down trehalose, a mushroom disaccharide, resulting in diarrhea on ingestion of mushrooms. The third category is absorption defects, as of glucose and galactose. These may be congenital or hereditary and are life-threatening to the infant. When acquired due to infectious gastroenteritis, absorption defects may be transitory. The treatment is elimination of all carbohydrates except fructose from the diet.

FAT DIGESTION AND ABSORPTION

Normal physiology

6

The normal daily adult diet contains 50 to 100 gm of fat, of which 90 per cent are triglycerides and the rest phospholipids and cholesterol esters. Triglycerides are esters of glycerol and long-chain saturated and unsaturated fatty acids. In contrast to the carbohydrates and proteins, triglycerides are practically insoluble in water, giving rise to special problems in their digestion and absorption. The first problem is their passage through the water layer separating them from the cells of the intestinal epithelium that must absorb them. The second problem, after absorption, is the transport of these fat molecules to the tissues where they are used or stored. The first problem is solved by means of bile salts, which form micelles. The second problem is solved by coupling of the lipids with proteins synthesized in the cells of the intestine, to form water-soluble lipoproteins.

In the human being, 96 per cent of ingested fat is efficiently digested. Therefore, excretion of more than 6 gm of fat a day is considered steatorrhea and indicates a defect in digestion and/or absorption.

Digestion and absorption of fats depend on the pancreas, which secretes lipolytic enzymes; on the liver, which secretes bile salts, necessary for the formation of micelles and consequent solubility; on the small intestine; and on the lymphatic system. The process takes place in steps. First, the intraluminal phase includes the breakdown of the fats into their component parts (lipolysis), the formation of micelles, and their diffusion across the aqueous barrier that covers the intestinal villi. The second, or membrane, phase consists of the passage of fats across the cellular membrane. The final, or intracellular, phase involves the resynthesis of fats, the formation of chylomicrons, and their transport to the lymphatic circulation. Digestion and absorption of fats are more complex and more difficult than for other components of the diet. Unabsorbed fats undergo no modification in structure while passing through distal segments of the gut. This explains why, clinically, poor absorption of fats with consequent steatorrhea is more apparent than poor absorption of carbohydrates, proteins, and other foods.

Lipolysis takes place in the upper part of the small intestine by the action of several lipolytic enzymes secreted by the pancreas. Lipase acts on the triglycerides, separating them into one molecule of beta-monoglyceride and two molecules of fatty acid. Cholesterol esterase acts on esterified cholesterol, separating it into free cholesterol and a fatty acid. Phospholipase converts lecithin into lysolecithin and fatty acids. Two gastrointestinal hormones play an important role in this stage of fat digestion: secretin and cholecystokinin-pancreozymin (CCK-PZ). Secretin keeps the pH of the lumen alkaline, to ensure optimum efficiency of the pancreatic enzymes. Its release is stimulated by hydrogen ions coming from the gastric juice, and it triggers pancreatic secretion of necessary amounts of sodium bicarbonate.

CCK-PZ, in turn, has a twofold action, as its name would indicate: It stimulates the pancreas to secrete its enzymes and at the same time causes the gallbladder to contract with consequent emptying of bile, rich in bile salts, into the intestine. This is most important in the micellar solubilization of fats. Colipase, another protein in pancreatic juice, helps lipase to stick to the surface of the oil droplets.

The products of lipolysis (fatty acids, monoglycerides, cholesterol, and lysolecithin) are only slightly soluble in water but are soluble in lipids. This makes it possible for them to cross through the epithelial cell membrane, which, like all cell membranes, is made up of lipids. Resistance to absorption of the products of lipolysis does not occur in the cellular membrane, but in the layer of water that normally covers the intestinal epithelium, as it covers many physiologic membranes, so that the principal value of bile salts in forming micelles with lipids is to overcome the resistance of this water layer.

The membrane stage consists of passage through the membrane of the epithelial cells. The process is passive. The micelle, once it has passed the water layer, liberates the fatty acids, monoglycerides, cholesterol, and lysolecithin into the cellular membrane, across which they then reach the interior of the cell. The bile salts are not absorbed there, but traverse the small intestine and are actively absorbed along the terminal part of the ileum.

The intracellular stage consists of the resynthesis of triglycerides, phospholipids, and cholesterol. Unlike the fats, carbohydrates and proteins are absorbed and arrive in the circulation broken into their component parts—monosaccharides and amino acids, respectively. The same does not happen with the lipids, which are resynthesized before entering the circulation. This is accomplished by enzymes present in the intestinal epithelial cells. After this resynthesis of lipids, a new problem arises: They must be made water-soluble in order to circulate and reach their final destination. The epithelial cells accomplish this also. They synthesize special globulins that combine with the lipids, forming chylomicrons. These leave the cells by some unknown process, penetrate the lacteal vessels located in the center of the intestinal villi, and thus reach the lymphatics, the thoracic duct, the superior vena cava, and the general circulation—in that order. The apoproteins that coat the chylomicrons potentiate the action of lipoprotein lipase, which coats the capillary surface and hydrolyzes the fats. Fatty acids are formed, bind to albumin, and then diffuse to cell membranes of tissues for uptake.

Bile salts, so important in absorption, are metabolic products of cholesterol. Their formation and partial excretion in the feces is important in the regulation of serum cholesterol levels. Cholesterol molecules, modified by hydroxylation of their steroid nucleus and breakdown of their lateral chain, are transformed into bile acids. Bile acids are molecules of completely different physicochemical properties, among which is the ability to allow lipids (including cholesterol itself) to become soluble in aqueous solutions. The bile acids are detergents with amphipathic properties; that is, they are soluble in water because they contain a hydrophilic area and are soluble in oil because they also contain a hydrophobic area. They tend to combine to form molecular complexes known as micelles. Micelles can incorporate the products of lipolysis, forming "mixed" micelles, and thus enable these products to be transported in an aqueous medium.

The liver synthesizes daily around 0.5 gm of primary bile acids (cholic and chenodeoxycholic acids), combines these with glycine and taurine, and secretes them actively through the bile ducts, from which they pass to the gallbladder, where they are concentrated and stored. There they remain between meals until the hormone cholecystokinin causes contraction of the gallbladder and expels them into the intestine, where they form mixed micelles with the products of lipolysis. These compounds are then transported across the water layer and into the intestinal epithelial cells. The bile salts travel along the small intestine and are passively absorbed in the jejunum and ileum in small amounts. They are largely absorbed by an active mechanism in the terminal ileum and reach the liver by means of the portal circulation.

Some bile salts reach the colon, where they are deconjugated and dehydroxylated by bacterial enzymes to become secondary bile acids: deoxycholic and lithocholic. The enterohepatic cycle is completed by the secretion of the bile salts again in the liver. The total quantity of bile salts in the body is 2 to 3 gm and circulates between the liver and the gut at the rate of two cycles per meal. The liver therefore secretes 12 to 18 gm of bile salts daily. The bile salts are not completely absorbed. Approximately 0.5 gm is lost in the feces in 24 hours and is replaced by an equal amount synthesized from cholesterol by the liver.

Bibliography

Borgstrom B: On the interactions between pancreatic lipase and colipase and the substrate, and the importance of bile salts. *J Lipid Res* 16:411, 1975

Gray GM: Mechanisms of digestion and absorption of food. In *Gastrointestinal Disease* (Sleisenger MH, Fordtran JS, eds), 2nd ed, pp 241–250. Philadelphia: Saunders, 1978

Hoffman AF: Fat absorption and malabsorption: Physiology, diagnosis and treatment. *Viewpoints Dig Dis* 9: No 4, Sept 1977

Westergaard H, Dietschy JM: Normal mechanisms of fat absorption. *Med Clin North Am* 58:1413, 1974

SUMMARY

Fats are normally handled very efficiently in the gastrointestinal tract, 96 per cent being digested and absorbed. This overall process depends on the pancreas, liver, small intestine, and lymphatic system and takes place in three phases. The first, or intraluminal phase, in the upper part of the small intestine, is lipolysis (breakdown of fat) by three pancreatic enzymes. Lipase breaks down triglycerides into beta-monoglyceride and two molecules of fatty acid; esterase separates esterified cholesterol into free cholesterol and a fatty acid; phospholipase converts lecithin into lysolecithin and fatty acids. Here two gastrointestinal hormones also act. Secretin maintains an alkaline pH and triggers pancreatic secretion of necessary sodium bicarbonate. Cholecystokinin-pancreozymin (CCK-PZ) stimulates the pancreas to release its enzymes and causes the gallbladder to contract and empty its bile into the intestine. The latter forms molecular complexes, or micelles, that incorporate the products of lipolysis. These complexes are soluble in both water and oil and therefore are able to cross the layer of water covering the epithelial cells of the gut.

The second, or membrane, phase begins with the micelles crossing the epithelial membrane, liberating fatty acids, monoglycerides, cholesterol, and lysolecithin into the interior of the cells. The bile salts, however, traverse the small intestine to be absorbed in the terminal ileum.

The third, or intracellular, phase consists of resynthesis of triglycerides, phospholipids, and cholesterol. They are made water-soluble by combining with newly synthesized globulins to form chylomicrons, which then penetrate the lacteal vessels and reach the lymphatics, thoracic duct, superior vena cava, and general circulation. The chylomicrons are coated with apoproteins that stimulate lipoprotein lipase to hydrolyze the fats, forming fatty acids that bind to albumin and diffuse to cell membranes for uptake.

Pathophysiology of the digestion and absorption of fats

7

The various steps in the normal digestion and absorption of fats may be disturbed, resulting in deficient absorption of both fats and fat-soluble compounds.

Pancreatic insufficiency

Exocrine pancreatic insufficiency occurs in cystic fibrosis and in the final stages of chronic pancreatitis, when most of the pancreatic parenchyma has been destroyed and what remains is insufficient to produce the necessary lipolytic enzymes—that is, when less than 10 per cent of normal production takes place. This is also seen in obstruction of the pancreatic duct and following total pancreatectomy. It results in deficient absorption of fats and fat-soluble vitamins, steatorrhea, malnutrition, deficient absorption of calcium, which forms soaps with the fats, osteomalacia, and sometimes tetany and hypomagnesemia. The clinical picture and diagnosis are described in Chapter 55. Treatment consists of diet with limited fats and added pancreatic enzymes by mouth to make up for the lipase deficiency.

Functional pancreatic insufficiency may result from inadequate stimulation by CCK-PZ because of damage of the intestinal mucosa where this hormone is secreted. It has been suggested that this mechanism contributes to the deficient absorption of fats in celiac sprue.

Hypersecretion of gastric acid

Some patients with gastrinoma, a tumor whose cells secrete gastrin, will have steatorrhea alone or with an especially severe ulcer syndrome (Zollinger-Ellison syndrome). This can be explained by hypersecretion of gastric acid in excess of the neutralizing ability of pancreatic bicarbonate secretion, thus lowering the pH of the duodenum. An acid medium prevents pancreatic enzymes from functioning properly and also interferes with the formation of micelles.

Insufficient bile salts

Steatorrhea can result from interference with the normal metabolism of bile acids. This happens especially when (1) there is bacterial overgrowth or (2) there is loss of bile salts. Normally the bacterial population in the small intestine is low: less than 10^3/ml. Bacteria become progressively more abundant from the duodenum to the terminal ileum. When intestinal movement is slow or stops (intestinal stasis), bacteria multiply 1 million times, producing an increase in dehydroxylation and deconjugation of bile salts. Because of their altered chemical and ionic structure, the bile salts are then unable to form normal mixed micelles and are absorbed passively in the proximal segments of the small intestine, resulting in incomplete digestion and absorption of fats and steatorrhea.

This is what occurs in patients with intestinal strictures, surgically produced blind loops, afferent loops that empty poorly, multiple jejunal diverticulosis, diabetic neuropathy, and scleroderma. Antibiotics can cut down the number of bacteria quite markedly and thus improve fat absorption. Unfortunately, this improvement is only temporary. Better results are obtained when the condition can be corrected surgically. The predominant bacteria are *Bacteroides,* coliforms, *Lactobacillus, Enterococcus,* and diphtheroids. Antibiotics most commonly used are tetracycline (Achromycin, Panmycin, others), ampicillin (Amcill, Omnipen, others), and kanamycin (Kantrex).

Decreased absorption of bile salts

Biliary acids may be lost in excessive amounts when the terminal ileum, their site of active absorption, has been surgically resected or when it is involved in pathology that interferes with its function. Passage through the colon causes choleretic diarrhea because they interfere with the transport of water and electrolytes in the mucosa (see Chapter 2). Their elimination in the feces reduces the total biliary acid content of the body. If the loss exceeds the liver's compensatory ability to synthesize them, steatorrhea inevitably results. The diarrhea produced by the action of the biliary acids on the colon may be corrected by giving cholestyramine, a chelating resin that sequesters these acids. Unfortunately, this treatment, although it cures the diarrhea, increases the fecal loss of biliary acids and may give rise to some degree of steatorrhea. This therapeutic problem may be resolved partially, at least, by substituting medium-chain fatty acids (commercially available) for the fats ordinarily eaten. Their caloric value is the same and they are more easily absorbed even in the absence of optimum concentrations of biliary acids.

Interference with transport of fat

The most important cause of poor fat absorption is interference with its transport into the interior of the epithelial cells. Transport depends on two things: the total area of intestinal mucosa and the functional capacity of its cells. If the lining of the small intestine were smooth, its surface would be about 3,300 sq cm, but because of its many folds, the villi that cover it, and the microvilli of these same intestinal cells, the total area is 600 times that, i.e., 2,000,000 sq cm. This explains the intestine's remarkable absorptive ability, and also why surgical removal of part of the intestine, and especially atrophy of the villi and microvilli in celiac sprue and other diseases, results in malabsorption. Another factor contributing to malabsorption is decreased function of the epithelial cells—in many cases, loss of their ability to re-esterify lipids. This is thought to be a possible cause of steatorrhea in Whipple's disease.

As noted, the formation of chylomicrons requires the synthesis of a beta-lipoprotein. If this does not occur, triglycerides accumulate in the epithelial cells and do not reach the lymphatics. This rare hereditary condition is called abetalipoproteinemia.

Clinical causes of steatorrhea

Clinically, the factors causing steatorrhea usually do not occur singly, but in various combinations. Thus, in celiac sprue, the area of absorption is decreased, the function of the epithelial cells is disturbed, and possibly there is deficient secretion of pancreatic enzymes as a result of decreased production of CCK-PZ by the damaged duodenal mucosa. Patients who have had partial gastrectomy with gastrojejunal anastomosis of the Billroth II type suffer from steatorrhea caused by too rapid passage of food from the stomach into the jejunum, resulting in inadequate stimulation of lipase secretion by the pancreas, insufficient mixing of the pancreatic enzymes with the food, too-rapid passage through the intestine, and excessive bacterial growth in the afferent loop when stasis occurs here. In addition, hypochlorhydria following surgery favors abnormal bacterial growth in the upper part of the small intestine and incomplete emptying of the gallbladder, resulting in deficient formation of micelles because of the rapid passage of foods into the jejunum with insufficient production of the hormone cholecystokinin (see Chapter 33).

Bibliography

Ament M, Shimoda S, Saunders D, et al: The pathogenesis of steatorrhea in three cases of small intestinal stasis syndrome. *Gastroenterology* 63:728, 1972

Isselbacher KJ, Scheig R, Plotkin GR, et al: Congenital beta-lipoprotein deficiency: An hereditary disorder involving a defect in the absorption and transport of lipids. *Medicine* 43:347, 1964

Lewis R, Gorbach S: Modification of bile acids by intestinal bacteria. *Arch Intern Med* 130:545, 1972

SUMMARY

Alterations of fat metabolism that cause disease

Stage altered	Mechanism	Disease
Lipolysis	Exocrine pancreatic insufficiency	Chronic pancreatitis; cystic fibrosis; obstruction of pancreatic duct
	Abnormal duodenal pH	Zollinger-Ellison syndrome
	Insufficient production of CCK-PZ	Abnormal intestinal mucosa
Formation of micelles	Insufficient bile salts	Biliary obstruction; ileal resection; ileal pathology; cholestyramine
Transport into epithelial cells	Changes in bile salts by bacterial action	Stasis, blind loop, afferent loop
	Decreased area of absorption	Intestinal resection
	Loss of normal function of epithelial cells	Celiac sprue; Whipple's syndrome

continued

Stage altered	Mechanism	Disease
Formation of chylomicrons	Deficient synthesis of beta-globulin	Abetalipoproteinemia
	Lymphatic pathology	Intestinal lymphangiectasia
Lymphatic circulation	Lymphatic obstruction	Cancer, lymphoma

DIGESTION AND ABSORPTION OF PROTEINS

Normal physiology

8

The normal human adult ingests 50 to 100 gm
of animal and vegetable protein daily. To this
must be added 35 to 130 gm of endogenous protein, which
reaches the intestinal lumen as digestive secretions rich in
enzymes, mucus, desquamated epithelial cells, and an unknown amount of plasma proteins. The daily fecal excretion
of proteins is 6 to 12 gm (1 to 2 gm of nitrogen), which indicates how efficient the digestion and absorption of proteins
are in a healthy individual.

Digestion of proteins

As in the case of carbohydrates, digestion of proteins takes
place by stages. The intraluminal stage involves the diges-

tive action of gastric pepsin and the proteolytic pancreatic enzymes trypsin, chymotrypsin, elastase, and carboxypeptidase. Pepsin acts in the acid medium of the stomach, converting proteins into large polypeptides. Its contribution to the total digestive process is small, since digestion hardly suffers at all in cases of gastric achylia or gastrectomy. The pancreatic enzymes are, however, truly important in the intraluminal stage.

The first stage is the activation of the proenzyme trypsinogen, which is changed to trypsin by enterokinase. Trypsin in turn activates other proteolytic enzymes. Trypsin, chymotrypsin, and elastase are endopeptidases. They attack internal peptide bonds while the carboxypeptidases remove carboxyl-terminal amino acids. The final products of this intraluminal stage are oligopeptides—small polypeptides containing six or fewer amino acid residues—as well as free amino acids.

The next stage in protein digestion takes place by means of peptide hydrolases located in the brush border (membrane) of the intestinal villi. The peptide hydrolases act preferably on oligopeptides, converting them into absorbable products: amino acids, dipeptides, and tripeptides. The digestion and absorption of dietary proteins are completed mainly in the upper small intestine, but part of this process may extend into the ileum.

Transport of
protein digestion products

There are two different mechanisms of transport for the products of protein digestion: amino acid transport and peptide transport. Both mechanisms are actively accomplished by carriers (interrelated but to some extent independent). Amino acids are transported by at least two distinct systems: one for neutral amino acids (e.g., leucine, phenylalanine, and threonine), and the other for basic amino acids (e.g., lysine, arginine, and cystine).

Amino acid constituents of dietary proteins are absorbed mostly as oligopeptides rather than as free amino acids. Most dipeptides and at least some tripeptides (but not larger oligopeptides) are transported by peptide carrier systems. Upon entering the enterocytes they undergo rapid hydrolysis by cytoplasmic peptide hydrolases. Only small quantities escape hydrolysis by these enzymes and enter the portal circulation as dipeptides. Eventually most products of protein digestion reach the portal circulation in the form of free amino acids.

Free amino acids are less readily absorbed from the intestine than are partially hydrolyzed proteins rich in di- and tripeptides. The more efficient absorption of di- and tripeptides holds practical importance. For patients who need protein and have trouble with absorption from the small intestine (cases of short intestine, extensive regional enteritis, tropical sprue, etc.), it's better to give easily digested proteins—for instance, casein, egg albumin, or hydrolyzed proteins containing mixtures of peptides and amino acids—than to give solutions of free amino acids. In addition to being more poorly absorbed, free amino acids are hypertonic and cause osmotic diarrhea.

Bibliography

Adibi SA: Intestinal phase of protein assimilation in man. *Am J Clin Nutr* 29:205, 1976

SUMMARY

The first, or intraluminal, stage of protein digestion involves in small degree gastric pepsin, but in much greater degree the pancreatic enzymes. Trypsinogen is changed by enterokinase to trypsin, which activates other pancreatic enzymes—chymotrypsin and elastase, both endopeptidases. Finally, the carboxypeptidases act. The results of this stage are the oligopeptides and free amino acids.

The second, or membrane, stage is carried out by the peptide hydrolases in the brush border of the intestinal villi, converting oligopeptides to absorbable free amino acids and di- and tripeptides. Most of this takes place in the upper small intestine but may extend into the ileum. Separate transport mechanisms exist for amino acids and peptides, and for neutral and basic amino acids. The greater part of proteins are absorbed as oligopeptides that are transported by a peptide carrier system into the portal circulation, where they are hydrolyzed to dipeptides and free amino acids.

Pathophysiology of the digestion and absorption of proteins

9

There is no clinical syndrome due to faulty digestion and absorption of peptides, in contrast to the well-known ones due to disturbed digestion of oligosaccharides. Congenital deficiencies of enterokinase and trypsin do, however, occur in children, interfering with the digestion and absorption of proteins and resulting in hypoproteinemia and edema. Also, it is believed that celiac sprue, described in Chapter 40, is due to the lack of a specific intestinal peptide hydrolase that normally would break down a toxic peptide occurring in gluten, which then accumulates in the intestinal cells of celiac patients.

Clinical pictures of malabsorption of amino acids are well known. These occur in all diseases with damage to the intes-

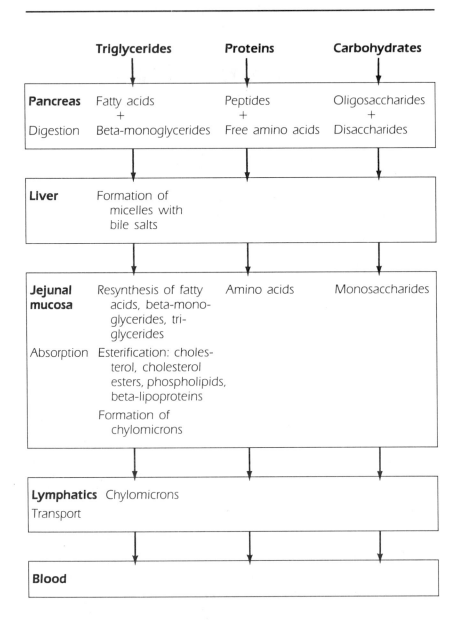

FIGURE 9-1 **General scheme of digestion of triglycerides, proteins, and carbohydrates**

tinal epithelium, such as celiac sprue, tropical sprue, and inflammatory diseases; after surgical reduction in length of the small intestine; and, to a moderate degree, in diseases of the pancreas. Here malabsorption of amino acids is accompanied by malabsorption of many other nutrients.

There are a number of rare hereditary diseases, not productive of diarrhea, that have in common a deficiency of one or more components of the amino acid transport system, both in the proximal loop of the kidney and in the intestine. These include Hartnup's disease, a defect in the transport of neutral amino acids; cystinuria, a defect in the transport of cystine and the basic amino acids lysine, arginine, and ornithine; the "blue diaper" syndrome, a defect in the transport of tryptophan; and a genetic defect in the absorption of methionine.

Figure 9-1 presents a comprehensive scheme of the digestion of triglycerides, proteins, and carbohydrates.

Bibliography

Freeman HJ, Kim YS: Digestion and absorption of protein. *Annu Rev Med* 29:99, 1978

Gray GM, Cooper HL: Protein digestion and absorption. *Gastroenterology* 61:535, 1971

Mathews DM: Memorial lecture: Protein absorption—then and now. *Gastroenterology* 73:1267, 1977

Mathews DM, Adibi SA: Peptide absorption. *Gastroenterology* 71:151, 1976

Silk DBA: Peptide absorption in man. *Gut* 15:494, 1974

PART II

THE PATIENT WITH DIARRHEA

Classification of diarrheas

10

Section A of Part I presented a pathophysiologic classification of diarrhea (see Tables 2-1, 2-2, and 2-3). Although this classification may help us to understand the mechanism of diarrhea and therefore to treat it appropriately, its diagnostic value is limited. Another classification, one based on anatomic findings, etiology, and symptomatology, is more useful in the empirical clinical setting.

TABLE 10-1

Acute diarrhea

Dietary indiscretions	Infestation	Drugs
Food intoxication	Food idiosyncrasy	Postinfection
Infection	Emotion	Allergy

continued

TABLE 10-1 _____

Chronic diarrhea

Organic (with organic lesions
in the digestive apparatus)

Specific locales

Rectum
  Inflammation
  Ulceration
  Tumor
  Fecal impaction

Colon
  Inflammation
  Ulceration
  Tumor
  Diverticulosis

Small intestine: without
malabsorption
  Inflammation
  Ulceration
  Stenosis
  Tumor
  Iatrogenic: radiation, medication

Small intestine: with malabsorp-
tion limited to one nutrient
  Lactose
  Other disaccharides
  Monosaccharides
  Lipids
  Others

Small intestine: with malabsorption of multiple nutrients
  Celiac sprue (gluten
  enteropathy)
  Tropical sprue
    Intestinal resection and short
    circuits
    Infection: regional enteritis,
    tuberculosis, nongranulomatous
    jejunitis, Whipple's disease
    Infestation: *Giardia lamblia,
    Ancylostoma duodenale,*

*Necator americanus,
Strongyloides stercoralis,
Coccidioides immitis,
Schistosoma mansoni*
Neoplasms
  Lymphoma
  Cancer
Collagen disease: scleroderma
Infiltrations: amyloidosis
Ischemia
Malnutrition
Iatrogenic
  Radiation
  Neomycin
Others
  Intestinal lymphangiectasia
  Eosinophilic gastroenteritis
  Hypogammaglobulinemia
  and dysgammaglobulinemia
  Carcinoid syndrome
  Dermatosis: herpetiform
  dermatitis, exfoliative
  dermatitis, eczema,
  erythrodermic psoriasis
  Syndrome of watery diarrhea,
  hypochlorhydria, and
  hypokalemia

Pancreas
  Exocrine pancreatic insufficiency
    Chronic pancreatitis
    Carcinoma
    Cystic fibrosis
    Resection
  Obstruction of the pancreatic duct
  Inactivation of pancreatic
  enzymes: Zollinger-Ellison
  syndrome

Specific locales

Liver and bile ducts
  Extrahepatic bile duct
  obstruction
  Intrahepatic cholestasis
  Deficient absorption of bile salts
  Deconjugation and dehydroxy-
  lation of bile salts

Stomach (subjected to surgery)
  Dumping syndrome
  Insufficient mixing
  Afferent loop
  Vagotomy

Functional (with no
demonstrable organic lesion)
  Psychogenic
  Endocrine

Method for studying the patient with diarrhea

11

Ordinarily diarrhea is a simple, self-limiting pathophysiologic distur-bance whose diagnosis and treatment present little problem. But not infrequently it is the symptom of a serious disease or is difficult to treat, posing a diagnostic and therapeutic chal-lenge to the physician. The mechanisms and causes of diar-rhea are so many and varied that a definite plan must be fol-lowed to minimize the chances of error and failure.

Acute diarrhea

The plan is simple when the diarrhea is acute. By definition, acute diarrhea is an illness of short duration either because it is self-limited with spontaneous recovery or because its cause is easily discovered and its treatment simple. In acute diarrhea, the diagnostic approach includes information as to the appearance of the stools, history of unwise eating or drinking, specific foods eaten, symptoms of infection, toxic and allergic reactions, medicines and other possible iatrogenic factors, emotional tension and conflicts, and epidemiologic data.

This history, along with the physical findings (which should include a rectal examination, inspection of the stool, and, if possible, a proctosigmoidoscopy) and the laboratory tests for pathogenic bacteria and parasites, clarifies the etiologic diagnosis of acute diarrhea in most cases. It is very useful to check for leukocytes in the stool smear. If they are numerous, this indicates a *Shigella* infection.

Chronic diarrhea

In chronic diarrhea, the problem is more difficult. Diagnosis requires a thorough knowledge not only of the pathophysiology of the syndrome and the pathology of the digestive tract but also of the various organs and systems whose malfunction can cause diarrhea. Many good methods have been described for diagnosis. In our experience, the following plan has given the best results:

1. History
   a. Information about the stools
   b. Information about defecation
   c. Review of the various segments and components of the digestive system (rectum, colon, small intestine, pancreas, liver, biliary tract, stomach)
   d. Information about intestinal malabsorption
   e. Information about organs and systems outside the digestive system
   f. Information about psychological tension and emotional conflicts
   g. Information about endocrine diseases
2. Physical examination
3. Inspection of the stool
4. Proctosigmoidoscopy

5. Routine laboratory work
   a. Complete stool examination, including culture for pathogenic organisms and search for ova and cysts of parasites
   b. Blood count, urinalysis, and blood chemistry
6. Routine X-ray studies
   a. Thorax
   b. Plain film of abdomen
   c. Barium enema
   d. Small bowel
7. Special tests as indicated by individual clinical problem
   a. Quantitative tests for fats and fecal nitrogen
   b. Lactose tolerance test
   c. D-Xylose test
   d. Schilling test (vitamin B_{12} absorption)
   e. Biopsy of small intestine
   f. Serum electrophoresis and immunoelectrophoresis
   g. Tests for exocrine pancreatic function
   h. Gastric secretory tests
   i. Other tests: breath, thyroid, adrenal, 5-hydroxy-indoleacetic acid excretion in urine, abdominal arteriography, pancreatography
   j. Colonoscopy
   k. Tests to evaluate metabolic and hydroelectrolytic consequences of diarrhea: serum proteins, calcium, phosphorus, magnesium, alkaline phosphatase, carotene, electrolytes, prothrombin time; X-ray of the skeleton.

The clinical history

12

The clinical history of every patient with diarrhea should be detailed and should include the present illness, a review of body systems, treatment to date, and past medical history. The following information is of special importance and should be gathered carefully.

Age

The most commonly seen causes of diarrhea in geriatric patients are laxative abuse, tumors of the colon, and diverticular disease. In young patients you should consider the irritable bowel syndrome, intestinal parasites, inflammatory bowel disease, lactose intolerance, and celiac sprue. It's unusual for an irritable bowel to start giving symptoms in elderly people.

Sex

Women suffer more often than men from an irritable bowel, hyperthyroidism, and radiation proctitis secondary to radiation therapy for cancer of the uterine cervix. Men suffer more than women from malignant tumors and diverticular disease of the colon.

Duration of the diarrhea

This information is very important. Diarrhea of more than two years' duration practically rules out malignant neoplasms. More likely diagnoses are irritable colon, lactose intolerance, inflammatory bowel disease, and malabsorption from whatever cause.

Course of symptoms

The course of the diarrhea gives valuable information. Irritable colon and nonspecific ulcerative colitis have an intermittent course with relapses and remissions. Patients with irritable colon have periods of diarrhea alternating with periods of constipation and normal stools. In ulcerative colitis there may be periods of constipation; rectal bleeding is the most characteristic symptom of this disease.

The stools

A study of the stools is of prime importance. Abnormal changes correspond to pathology and malfunction of the digestive organs and may furnish important clues, helpful in arriving at a diagnosis. Whenever possible, inspect the feces. Sometimes this is not possible, or sometimes stool samples collected or obtained by rectal examination give only partial or misleading information and are not typical. Therefore, patients should be carefully questioned on this subject. A patient may dislike looking at his stools and be unable to give exact information. In this case, a list of questions on the subject should be handed to the patient; he is told to observe carefully and to report in detail at the next visit.

Normal stools

Normal stools are pasty, smooth, and cylindrical. They measure 15 to 30 cm in length in adults and are 2 to 4 cm in diameter. They weigh between 75 and 150 gm. They are made up of 25 to 30 per cent solids and 70 per cent water. Bacteria constitute one-third of the solids; the rest consist of intestinal secretions and unabsorbed enzymes, desquamated epithelial cells, and undigested foods. The color of the stool is due to fecal urobilin (stercobilin) formed by the action of intestinal bacterial enzymes on bilirubin secreted in the bile. The odor is sui generis and comes from aromatic substances such as indole and skatole, which are produced by the decomposition of proteins in the intestine and are also derived directly from the amino acid tryptophan.

Find out from the patient the number, shape, consistency, volume, color, and odor of the stools and the presence of abnormal components: undigested food, mucus, blood, pus, macroscopic parasites, and fat globules.

Number, volume, and fluidity

These characteristics depend especially on the degree of irritability of the distal colon and, to a lesser extent, on the fecal volume that reaches this segment. Very frequent, small, liquid stools are seen particularly in diseases where there is marked irritability of the distal colon and rectum: inflammatory and ulcerative diseases, tumors of the rectum and sigmoid, and, of course, irritable bowel.

Numerous liquid stools of large volume are seen when large amounts of fluid reach the intestinal lumen, as in cholera and choleriform syndromes, such as bacterial enteritis. In cholera, the liquid feces contain small flecks of mucus, which have given rise to the term rice-water stools.

Slightly softened stools are not necessarily abnormal, but are more likely to occur in people with irritable bowel. If the functional disturbance of the colon becomes more severe, or if there are inflammatory changes, the stools become frankly liquid or are expelled in semisolid, friable segments that promptly disintegrate.

Villous adenoma of the distal colon and rectum is another condition that can be responsible for copious liquid stools (with volumes up to 4 liters a day) and consequent hydro-electrolytic imbalance.

Whenever the colon is not abnormally irritable, the feces are stored and, consequently, subjected to further absorption of their water content for longer periods of time. This results in fewer, larger, and more solid stools, as seen in diarrhea originating in disturbances of the small intestine.

In patients with malabsorption syndrome the stools are typically bulky, pale, pasty, foamy, greasy, with a fetid odor, and they usually float in water. They may, however, be liquid, especially during flare-ups, while at other times they may appear normal even though chemical examination will show the presence of steatorrhea. The large volume of the stool is due not only to the presence of unabsorbed food but also to the capacity of the distal colon, which is healthy, to hold large amounts of feces without triggering the defecation urge.

The stools in pancreatic insufficiency of whatever origin greatly resemble those of malabsorption. Fat may be seen as drops of oil in the stool.

Color

The color of the stools depends to some extent on the diet. Large amounts of milk turn the stools light yellow. If the diet is largely meat, they are dark brown. Spinach and other vegetables rich in chlorophyll produce green stools, while beets lend their red color. Large amounts of chocolate may produce a dark, wine-red, or brown color that resembles melena.

Endogenous factors may affect the color of the stools. In steatorrhea, stools are pale. In biliary obstruction or cholestasis, the color is even paler. Excessive amounts of bile impart a yellow or green color. Hemorrhage, if high up in the digestive tract, causes melena—black, tarry stools; dark red if they are quickly expelled.

Some medications affect the color of the stool: carbon makes it black; bismuth turns it a dark gray; and iron produces a greenish black.

Odor

The odor of the stools gives information to the alert clinician. Like color, odor is influenced by various factors. An excess of proteins aids putrefaction and makes the stools more fetid. An abundance of vegetables decreases the odor. On a milk diet the odor practically disappears. Endogenous factors also influence odor: A sour, pungent, or fetid smell accompanies malabsorption; in acute enteritis the smell is very foul. In cholera, the stool smells like sperm, and in carcinoma of the colon it may sometimes carry a "gangrenous" odor.

Food residues

Normal stools do not contain undigested food unless the diet has excessive amounts of residues such as tomatoes, corn, or peas. These residues are more easily seen if the stools are liquid. The habit of swallowing large pieces of unchewed food may also be responsible. Stools with much undigested food passed very soon after eating suggest that the distance between the stomach and the rectum has become shortened either by extensive resection of the intestine, short circuits, or gastroileal anastomosis, or by gastrocolic fistulae. Stools containing undigested food occur also in cases of pancreatic insufficiency.

Mucus and pus

The presence of mucus doesn't necessarily indicate an inflammatory process. Large amounts of mucus occur in the stools of patients with functional diseases of the colon. A nervous disorder of the colon, which for some unknown reason has become less common, is characterized by a large amount of fecal mucus and has been named mucous colitis. Sometimes the material passed is liquid, but at other times it may look like false membranes or pieces of intestinal lining. This alarms the patient: He thinks he's passing pieces of his intestine or enormous worms. Laxatives and irritating enemas are common causes of excessive mucus production. A rare disease, colitis cystica profunda, may also cause excessive amounts of mucus.

Mucus is accompanied by pus and blood in inflammatory and neoplastic conditions. When you find this combination, suspect amebic, bacillary, or nonspecific ulcerative colitis or carcinoma of the colon or rectum.

Although the mucus is generally produced in the colon, it may come from inflammatory processes in the small intestine. Consider this possibility if the mucus is colored green by bilirubin or if it is well mixed with more or less liquid feces.

In pseudomembranous colitis, described in Chapter 34, pieces of fibrinous membrane are expelled and the patients describe them as pieces of intestinal mucosa.

Blood

Blood in the stools is a most important indication of the presence of an organic lesion in the digestive tract. Its color depends on the site of bleeding and on how quickly it passes through the gastrointestinal tract. If the bleeding occurs in the upper part, it undergoes enzymatic action and becomes black (melena) unless it is passed very rapidly through the intestines, in which case it is wine-red, like blood arising from the small intestine and proximal colon. Fresh blood indicates a lesion in the distal colon, rectum, or anus. The most frequent causes of this are anal fissures, hemorrhoids, ulcerative inflammatory lesions, benign and malignant tumors, and inflamed diverticula. Blood mixed with mucus and pus comes from ulcerated inflammatory lesions or neoplasms.

Parasites

The following parasites may be seen easily and identified macroscopically in the stools: *Ascaris lumbricoides, Trichuris (Trichocephalus)*, pinworms, *Uncinaria (Necator, Ancylostoma)*, and tapeworms. Although these parasites may be expelled in a diarrheal stool, they may have no etiologic connection with the diarrhea.

Visible fat

Visible fat is a sign of steatorrhea unless the patient is taking oily laxatives. It's recognized from the special shine on the surface of the stools or from drops of fat that float in the water of the toilet. Steatorrhea is the common denominator of an important group of diseases of malabsorption. If the steatorrhea is of pancreatic origin, actual leakage of oil from the anus may occur.

Normal stools are slightly heavier than water; they sink. If they float, they contain abnormally high amounts of a lighter material—i.e., fat or gas. Feces that float have been considered typical of steatorrhea of either intestinal or pancreatic origin. Recently, however, studies have shown that stools in steatorrhea do not contain enough fat to cause them to float. Their buoyancy can be explained by the presence of gas, especially methane. Most stools that float are not due to steatorrhea, despite what was previously believed.

Information about defecation

The time of defecation, accompanying pain, urgency, tenesmus, and relation to eating, kinds of food eaten, and psychic factors are all important.

Periodicity

Some diarrheal syndromes have a characteristic time of defecation. When the trouble is in the small intestine, diarrhea is often predominantly nocturnal. This is especially typical of diabetic diarrhea. Nervous diarrhea rarely wakes patients at night. Patients with irritable colon wake early in the morning with an urgent desire to defecate. In irritable colon and in nearly all cases of inflammatory bowel disease, stools tend to occur immediately after meals, as if the nervous or humoral mechanism that normally stimulates the colon to action when food arrives in the stomach or duodenum had been speeded up. This was formerly attributed to a gastrocolic reflex; now cholecystokinin has been proposed as the hormone responsible.

Pain

Pain may precede, accompany, or follow defecation, and may occur in the lower abdomen or its left lower quadrant. Most commonly it consists of cramping, and it precedes and is relieved by defecation. It may vary from mild cramping to severe colic. Pain during and after defecation suggests that the colonic disturbance is not merely functional but organic. Pelvic peritonitis may cause diarrhea from extrinsic and centripetal irritation of the rectum. Here the pain is in the lower abdomen and pelvis, is continuous, and gets worse with any movement of the abdomen or its contents. But instead of alleviating the pain, defecation succeeds only in making it worse.

Urgency

Like pain, urgency indicates increased irritability of the rectum and distal colon, which contract vigorously on the arrival of fecal matter.

Tenesmus

This is a symptom of rectal spasm and indicates pathology of the rectum. It occurs typically in dysentery, that is, in amebic, bacterial, or nonspecific ulcerative proctocolitis, as well as in other conditions that involve the rectum, such as lymphogranuloma venereum and benign and malignant tumors. Tenesmus is significant in diarrheal diseases since it indicates that the rectum is involved.

The need to defecate shortly after eating arises in patients with irritable colon or inflammatory bowel disease. Two rare causes are gastrocolic fistula and a short bowel secondary to resection or surgical bypassing of the small intestine. In these conditions the stools contain undigested, recently ingested food (lientery).

Relation to physical activity

When the colon is inflamed, exercise may provoke a diarrheal stool. In chronic ulcerative colitis, when the distal colon has become a rigid tube lacking the muscular strength to contain the feces, even shifting position may cause an urge to empty the bowels.

Relation to certain foods

The patient with chronic diarrhea, influenced by a multitude of cultural prejudices, tends to attribute his symptoms to certain foods. The list grows longer all the time. Thus, many taboos originate; they're often not effectively counteracted by the physician. Patients blame their diarrhea on a great variety of foods which are generally quite inoffensive. In some cases, however, the patient is right.

Milk, especially, may cause diarrhea due to idiosyncrasy or, more frequently, to lactase deficiency, a widespread condition. It was common to see diarrhea develop shortly after patients were put on a milk diet for the treatment of peptic ulcer. When a sudden increase in lactose in the diet exceeds the capacity to digest it, diarrhea, which may be explosive, results. Lactose intolerance may also appear following an intestinal infection, probably because these diseases damage the intestinal epithelium, resulting in an acquired, transient lactase deficiency.

Other foods that may cause diarrhea are those containing gluten, a food component which affects people with celiac sprue (gluten-induced enteropathy).

Relation to psychic factors

This is universal. It has been noted and described by poets, writers, and historians. It is an integral part of the folklore of all nations and has acquired scientific standing through experimental work on animals and humans. Still, the fact that diarrhea follows emotional reactions does not establish it as being purely functional. To be content with this diagnosis without ruling out organic causes does injustice to the patient, because any organic disease may show this relation between psychological factors and diarrhea. It is imperative to rule out concomitant organic lesions in all patients with apparently functional, psychogenic diarrhea.

Review of the various segments and components of the digestive system

After obtaining all the information possible about the appearance of the stools and other characteristics of the diarrhea, methodically review the normal and pathologic physiology of each part of the organs that make up the digestive system. In this way essential information, necessary to a correct diagnosis, is gathered, amplified, and checked. The exact order in which these data are gathered is not important, so long as the whole field is covered.

- ☐ *Rectum.* Check for mucus and fresh blood; tenesmus and urgency; pain.
- ☐ *Colon.* Check for mucus and fresh blood; urgency; pain in the lower quadrants of the abdomen.
- ☐ *Small intestine.* Check for periumbilical pain and abdominal distention; fistulae; previous surgery.
- ☐ *Malabsorption syndrome.* Lactose intolerance is suggested by acid diarrheal stools, anal burning, borborygmi, and flatulence. Steatorrhea is suggested by bulky, pale, fetid, greasy, foamy stools that float. Other indirect evidence of possible malabsorption are nutritional symptoms and signs such as weight loss, retarded growth, weakness, glossitis, stomatitis, tetany, bone pain, paresthesias, hemorrhages, hypoproteinemic edema, and peripheral neuropathy.
- ☐ *Pancreas.* Check for the presence of pain; diabetes mellitus; steatorrhea.
- ☐ *Liver and biliary system.* Check for jaundice; pruritus; symptoms of liver failure.
- ☐ *Stomach.* Ask about a history of gastric surgery.

Information about organs and systems outside the digestive system

In the classification of diarrheas (Chapter 10), we have seen that diarrhea, though it involves the intestine, may be caused by organs or systems outside the digestive tract. It's advisable to check these completely and methodically.

Information about psychic tension and emotional conflicts

One of the most common chronic diarrheas is nervous diarrhea—functional disturbances of the intestine in whose etiology psychological factors play an important role. It is necessary to identify these factors. Diagnosis of this type of diarrhea cannot be made simply by ruling out organic lesions and functional disturbances of other origins.

The task is thus to identify symptoms of emotional tension, to uncover emotional conflicts, to establish a correlation between these conflicts and the onset of symptoms, and to get an overall picture of the patient's character and his psychological difficulties. One would like to delegate this task to a psychoanalyst, who is able to take the necessary time during long and frequent sessions. However, such a profound and extensive study is usually not necessary. Of course, there are patients whose psychological problems are so severe that they need extensive psychiatric exploration. Such patients should not be handled by a physician who has not had psychiatric training, but referred to a psychiatrist.

Actually it isn't as difficult as it may seem at first to handle the less severe cases. A knowledge of human nature is, of course, basic, but above all you must establish a rapport with the patient and be interested in knowing and understanding him as a human being. Then use common sense in interpreting and correlating the clinical data with the patient's emotional makeup. The information you gather, analyze, and synthesize does not need to be as profound as that required by a psychiatrist, nor is it necessary to get a complete psychiatric history during the first interview. The technique consists in developing an ability to study the patient psychologically during the history taking, the physical examination, and during later office calls. This can improve your powers of observation regarding nonverbal communication and emotional language and enable you to include these observations as an essential part of the clinical history. View the patient as a whole and encourage him to express his thoughts, ideals, frustrations, and conflicts. This should become part of the clinical workup. The spontaneous tendency of many patients to relate their symptoms to life situations and problems should be encouraged. Interviews following this plan will last a few minutes longer. But these extra minutes early in the course of therapy will save hours and weeks of effort, expense, and suffering that result from misdiagnosis and incorrect treatment.

Physical signs that reveal emotional tension should be looked for: wide-open staring eyes; cold, wet palms, sometimes trembling; restlessness; frequent changes in position; drumming with the fingers; rhythmic foot movements; inability to sit still; tics, sweating; need to light a cigarette. At other times these may be only subjective: anxiety, fear, restlessness, internal trembling, uneasiness, an impulse to run away, phobias, and compulsions of various kinds.

Functional disturbances of the colon may coincide with, and probably are expressions of, emotional conflicts. The most frequent conflicts are hostility, fear, insecurity, and guilt. It is important to uncover these emotions. Often the patient is eager to confide in his doctor. With a show of interest on your part, the patient will spontaneously relate incidents of his life and point out their relationship to his illness. If you, by means of *nonverbal communication,* let the patient know that what he is saying is important, the patient will continue to confide in you, revealing many things of great value to the diagnosis. At times it may be necessary to refer to an emotional conflict the patient has mentioned; to express interest by means of a gesture; to repeat a key word; to question gently; to encourage. Usually, then, the patient will speak freely and willingly of his experiences and repressed emotions. In these modern times we live what has been correctly termed a "conspiracy of silence." Modern industrial society is made up of people who have, to a large extent, lost their identity and their ability to communicate. The physician is one of the few human beings who still listens and tries to understand others. An atmosphere of understanding and sincere interest, free from disapproval or criticism, is ideal for the tense patient who is overwhelmed by his problems. It allows him to express himself freely, encouraged by a sympathetic listener. This not only is the best way to understand the patient but is of great value therapeutically.

Information about endocrine diseases

Various endocrine diseases present diarrhea as one of their important symptoms. Other symptoms may be minimized or overlooked by the patient. Therefore, it's routinely necessary to question the patient closely with these other conditions in mind. This is important in all cases of chronic diarrhea.

Diarrhea occurs in hyperthyroidism. In addition to its chronicity, it is particularly resistant to dietary and symptomatic treatment. Other symptoms to look for are nervousness, palpitations, sweating, tremors, and loss of weight in spite of a normal or high caloric diet. Hyperthyroidism should be ruled out in all cases of chronic diarrhea.

In chronic adrenal insufficiency, diarrhea is accompanied by anorexia, asthenia, skin and mucous membrane pigmentation, and weight loss.

Visceral neuropathy, as a complication of diabetes mellitus, is hard to miss. The patient not only has the very special characteristic diarrhea, described in Chapter 58, but is generally a diabetic of long standing, usually with several complications, including peripheral neuropathy. It is important to investigate other clinical findings of autonomic neuropathy to support the diagnosis of diarrhea of diabetic origin. These findings include abnormal sweating, bladder atony, sexual impotence, and postural hypotension.

Loss of weight

Not all chronic diarrhea is accompanied by loss of weight. The weight remains constant in irritable colon unless the patient restricts his food intake. Likewise, weight is unaffected in inflammatory disease of colon and rectum unless there is loss of protein in the blood and pus or the patient restricts his food intake. On the other hand, there may be marked weight loss in patients with malabsorption, hyperthyroidism, inflammatory disease of the small bowel, or malignant neoplasm.

Fever

Fever in a patient with diarrhea suggests infectious disease. Crohn's disease of the small intestine or colon, intestinal tuberculosis, nonspecific ulcerative colitis, invasive amebiasis, and lymphoma of the intestine are some of the diseases to be considered.

Past history

The following information should be sought routinely, since it is most important in making the etiologic diagnosis.

Eating habits

Bolting food and eating irregularly have been considered responsible for functional digestive disorders, including functional diarrhea. The true etiologic significance of these habits is difficult to evaluate, since tense individuals tend toward these habits. Their nervous tension, rather than their habits, may be the real cause of diarrhea.

Alcoholism

Abuse of alcoholic beverages may be the cause of the diarrhea. Tactful questioning of the patient generally establishes the relation between bouts of drinking and onset of the diarrheal episodes.

Medications

A growing number of drugs in use today may cause chronic diarrhea. It is imperative, therefore, to find out what drugs the patient is taking. Some common culprits are:

Antacids containing magnesium (Gaviscon, Maalox, many others)
Antibiotics: clindamycin (Cleocin) and lincomycin (Lincocin) especially, but also ampicillin, tetracyclines, etc.
Thyroid hormone (Proloid, Synthroid, others)
Potassium chloride (K-Lor, Kay Ciel, others)
Bile salts
Colchicine
Phenylbutazone (Butazolidin)
Indomethacin (Indocin)
Chemotherapeutic agents.

Surgical history

Many surgical procedures can interfere with the normal physiology of digestion, with resulting diarrhea. The most important are:

Gastric resection
Gastroenterostomy

Vagotomy

Resection of the small bowel or colon

Intestinal bypass procedures

Any laparotomy, if followed by adhesions causing incomplete intestinal obstruction, dilated loops, and bacterial overgrowth.

Other pathologic history

Many coexisting or past diseases can furnish the clue to the diagnosis of a chronic diarrhea:

Infections and infestations: tuberculosis, shigellosis, amebiasis, giardiasis, helminthiasis

Chronic diarrhea in childhood: celiac disease, milk intolerance, carbohydrate intolerance

Allergy

Psychological abnormalities

Dermatitis

Pancreatitis

Diabetes mellitus

Peptic ulcer (Zollinger-Ellison syndrome)

Hyperparathyroidism (multiple endocrine adenomatosis, possibly including a gastrinoma or vasoactive intestinal polypeptide-secreting tumor, also called vipoma).

Bibliography

Deutsch F: Associative anamnesis. *Psychoanal Q* 8:354, 1939

Levitt MD, Duane WC: Floating stools—flatus versus fat. *N Engl J Med* 286:973, 1972

Lisansky ET, History taking and interviewing. *Mod Treat* 6:656, 1969

Chapters 12 and 13 are summarized in Chapter 14.

The physical examination

Habitus

13

Initial inspection frequently yields more helpful information regarding etiology than does the rest of the physical examination. Such is the case with hyperthyroidism, the diagnosis of which is strongly suggested by exophthalmos, bright, staring eyes, hyperkinesis, and enlarged thyroid gland. An emaciated state may suggest sprue or Addison's disease, especially the latter if there is also brown pigmentation. Loss of weight, anemia, and malnutrition are visible physical signs pointing toward organic diarrheal diseases. Jaundice indicates the presence of hepatic or biliary disease.

The physical signs of psychic tension were listed in Chapter 12.

Skin

Every patient with diarrhea should have his skin carefully examined. Skin pigmentation is typical of Addison's disease but can also be seen in hyperthyroidism, pellagra, hemochromatosis, and cirrhosis of the liver (particularly biliary cirrhosis). It is also observed in patients suffering from malabsorption syndrome.

Pigmentation is associated with intestinal polyposis in Peutz-Jeghers syndrome, which is inherited in an autosomal dominant pattern with a high degree of penetrance. The polyposis results from the growth of multiple adenomas along the intestinal tract. Malignant degeneration is not seen in small intestinal polyps but does occur in polyps in the colon. The pigmentation takes the form of melanin macules in the face, fingers, palms, and oral mucosa.

Skin hemorrhages may be the result of prolongation of prothrombin time caused by liver failure, biliary tract obstruction, or intestinal malabsorption. The last two conditions interfere with the absorption of vitamin K.

Pellagra is characterized by erythema of the exposed parts: dorsa of the hands, bridge of the nose, and the neck. Hyperkeratosis, desquamation, and fissures follow the acute erythematous stage. Other cutaneous signs of avitaminosis are angular stomatitis and cheilosis (fissuring and dry scaling of the vermilion of the lips and angles of the mouth) associated with glossitis in patients with malabsorption syndrome.

Dull and brittle, or fine, silky, prematurely gray hair is frequently seen in malnourished patients or those with malabsorption syndrome. In children, hypertrichosis of the extremities may often accompany malnutrition.

Convex nails are seen in all types of steatorrhea and in regional enteritis. Concave nails occur in iron deficiency. Hypoalbuminemia causes transverse white marks (leukonychia) similar to those seen in chronic diseases of the liver. Malabsorption patients may have brittle nails with longitudinal striae. The nails tend to break at the edges (onychorrhexis). Hyperthyroidism commonly causes separation of the nail from the nail bed (onycholysis), especially on the ring finger.

Acanthosis nigricans is a melanin hyperpigmentation with papillomatous hypertrophy that occurs in the skin of the axillae, sides of the neck, perineum, genitalia, internal surface of the thighs, face, flexural folds, and around the umbilicus and anus. The mucous membranes of the mouth and genitalia may be pigmented and there may be warty growths and papillomas. Hyperkeratosis of the palms and soles may be associated. This condition is associated with adenocarcinomas of the digestive tract in 95 per cent of cases. In 20 per cent of these cases the acanthosis nigricans precedes other clinical signs of the malignant tumor by up to six years. It's important to differentiate this from a benign prepubertal pigmentation and from pseudoacanthosis nigricans of obese women—neither of which is clinically important.

Pyoderma gangrenosum is a confluent pustular eruption with marked tendency to extend and coalesce. It begins as small nodules, vesicles, or furuncles that grow, ulcerate, and coalesce, forming large areas surrounded by a purple undermined border. This is a complication of chronic inflammatory bowel disease. Other complications may be erythema nodosum and nonspecific dermatoses such as erythemas, pustules, acneiform lesions, urticaria, leg ulcers, and lesions resembling dermatitis herpetiformis.

Systemic sclerosis, or scleroderma, is characterized by thickening and condensation of collagen with secondary atrophy. The muscular layers of the intestinal wall and the skin are the areas most often affected, as described in Chapter 46. The skin lesions are seen especially on the hands and to a lesser extent on the face, neck, trunk, arms, and legs. The skin is thickened, lustrous, and waxy with subcutaneous induration. Often the pigmentation may be diffuse or freckle-like combined with areas of depigmentation. Telangiectasis, ungual dystrophy, ulceration of the fingertips, and Raynaud's disease may also appear.

Dermatitis herpetiformis is a chronic skin disease characterized by small, itchy vesicles on the extensor surfaces of the body. It often concurs with histologic and physiopathologic changes in the small intestine similar to celiac sprue, and sometimes with diarrhea and steatorrhea. Finding dermatitis herpetiformis in a patient with chronic diarrhea should suggest these diseases.

Patients suffering from malignant carcinoid of the intestine may present with a cyanotic blush of the face that is spontaneous or stimulated by emotion, ingestion of alcoholic beverages, abdominal palpation, or enemas. With time the vasodilation becomes permanent and the face develops a violaceous color.

Finally, intestinal neoplasms may metastasize to the skin and form subcutaneous nodules.

Eyes

Exophthalmos and other signs of hyperthyroidism are evident on inspection. Uveitis can indicate the presence of chronic inflammatory bowel disease. Retinitis pigmentosa may occur with abetalipoproteinemia. In addition to concentric narrowing of the visual fields, irregular, dark pigment stains occur in the periphery of the retina.

Mouth

The buccal and lingual mucous membranes may be affected by vitamin deficiency as seen in the malabsorption syndrome. Reddening, ulceration, swelling, and burning of the tongue and fissures of the mouth (angular cheilosis) are common clinical signs.

Brown pigmentation of the lips may be the first sign of Addison's disease. It is seen also in Peutz-Jeghers syndrome. Here it has a different distribution, occurring around the lips, on the buccal mucous membrane, and around the eyes and nose.

Neck

These signs in the neck may be related to diarrhea: enlargement of the thyroid gland and enlargement of the cervical lymph nodes from infection (tuberculosis) or from neoplasms (metastasis, lymphomas), and also in Whipple's disease.

Thorax

Examination of the thorax may give important diagnostic information regarding diarrhea: signs of pulmonary tuberculosis; signs and symptoms of bronchiectasis, which is part of the picture in cystic fibrosis of the pancreas or following hypogammaglobulinemia, with or without steatorrhea; pulmonary metastasis of neoplasms responsible for the diarrhea; and mediastinal lymphadenopathy in lymphomas.

Abdomen

Examination of the abdomen is particularly important in patients with chronic diarrhea and should be done carefully and in logical sequence. Inspection may reveal the following:

- □ Metastatic nodules from abdominal neoplasms
- □ Mottled pigmentation from frequent application of heat to relieve pain
- □ Collateral venous network secondary to portal hypertension
- □ Umbilical hernia of recent appearance suggesting ascites, abdominal tumor, or other causes of increased intra-abdominal pressure
- □ Flaccidity and wet rag sign of the abdominal wall indicate recent weight loss of considerable amount
- □ Postoperative scars
- □ Asymmetry and swellings caused by tumors or obstructed and distended intestinal loops
- □ Visible peristalsis from intestinal obstruction.

Superficial and deep palpation is of great importance. Resistance to palpation suggests underlying peritoneal irritation. Palpable descending and sigmoid colon results from spastic contraction, characteristic of the irritable bowel syndrome. It is not only palpable but also painful in diverticulitis or acute inflammation. Tumors of the colon are relatively easy to detect by palpation when they are located in the cecum or ascending colon. Inflamed loops of the ileum are found in regional enteritis and intestinal tuberculosis.

Palpation discloses changes outside the digestive system:

□ Changes in the liver: increased size, hardening and sharpening of the border in cirrhosis, very hard and nodular surface in metastatic carcinoma
□ Splenomegaly
□ Fistulas: chronic intra-abdominal inflammatory processes, especially regional enteritis
□ Ascites: hepatic disease and portal hypertension, tuberculous peritonitis, or peritoneal carcinomatosis.

Percussion is helpful in revealing tympanites in celiac sprue; shifting dullness of the flanks from free ascites; localized dullness from walled-off ascites; and dullness due to tumors and enlarged abdominal organs.

Auscultation of the abdomen should be done in all patients. Those with chronic diarrhea may have the following:

□ Hyperperistalsis, causing rapid transit through the intestines in many functional and organic diarrheal diseases
□ Signs of mechanical intestinal obstruction
□ Vascular bruits from stenotic abdominal arteries.

When diarrhea is caused by functional derangements of the colon, examination of the abdomen does not give positive signs of much diagnostic value. Sometimes, however, palpation of the cecum may produce borborygmi from the accumulation of liquid feces and gas in this segment. There is tenderness of the intestinal loops on deep pressure.

In patients with malabsorption, especially those with celiac sprue, the abdomen is frequently enlarged. This varies from a slight convexity, surprising in a patient who has lost much weight, to frank distention.

Regional enteritis is another disease with chronic diarrhea that yields significant findings on palpation. Fistulae opening through the abdominal wall may be seen, and thickened parts of the intestinal wall, forming adhesions and lumps, may be felt as thickened, painful loops or as frank masses. These findings are not always present in this disease. One may be surprised to find nothing on abdominal examination, even when the intestine is extensively inflamed.

Extremities

The hands

You can tell a great deal simply by shaking hands with the patient. A flaccid, cold, wet palm that gives hardly any pressure and is quickly withdrawn belongs to a patient with an anxiety neurosis. Restless, tobacco-stained fingers identify a heavy smoker, and bitten nails suggest worry or emotional anguish. A very strong handshake that practically breaks the bones suggests one type of defense a patient may use to overcome his anxieties. Fine, rapid tremor and damp, warm, fine skin suggest hyperthyroidism, while contracture of the palmar fascia identifies the patient as a chronic alcoholic. Occasionally, clubbed fingers may lead you to reconsider a diagnosis of nervous diarrhea; a more thorough investigation results in a diagnosis of regional enteritis. Clubbed fingers are also found in nonspecific ulcerative colitis and in malabsorption syndromes.

Pulse and blood pressure

The pulse is rapid in the anxious patient. A vagotonic patient with functional digestive disorders may have bradycardia. In active, nonspecific ulcerative colitis, the pulse is said to be disproportionately fast. The rate depends principally on the degree of fever, the amount of intoxication, and disturbances in hemodynamic and electrolyte balance caused by the disease.

Blood pressure should be taken with the patient lying down and standing up. Diseases accompanied by chronic diarrhea tend to cause low blood pressure, a finding explained by the malnutrition and the constant loss of liquids and electrolytes. Orthostatic hypotension is particularly noticeable in those patients whose diarrhea is secondary to an autonomic neuropathy (diabetes mellitus).

Edema

In patients with chronic diarrhea, edema is due to hypoproteinemia. Hypoproteinemia in turn may be caused by losing excessive amounts of protein in the stool (protein-losing enteropathy, intestinal lymphangiectasia, extensive inflammatory processes of the intestine, celiac sprue); deficient synthesis of protein in disease of the liver; or, less commonly, malnutrition. It may occur also in pancreatic insufficiency and deficient absorption of amino acids.

Arthritis

Arthritis in association with chronic diarrhea is seen in patients with chronic nonspecific ulcerative colitis, Crohn's disease, collagen disease, lymphoma, and Whipple's disease.

Circulatory disturbances

Raynaud's disease should suggest systemic sclerosis (scleroderma) as the cause of the diarrhea. Peripheral arterial insufficiency, either from arteriosclerosis or arteritis, but especially the latter, may give the diagnostic clue in cases of obscure abdominal symptoms.

Neurologic examination of the patient may reveal peripheral polyneuropathy from lack of thiamine, and subacute combined degeneration of the spinal cord from vitamin B_{12} deficiency.

Rectal examination

A rectal examination should be done on all patients. This axiom is particularly important in patients with diarrhea. Omitting such a simple part of the physical examination continues to be a source of unpardonable error.

Position

The best position is usually Sims's: Have the patient lie on his left side with the buttocks on the edge of the examining table, the body in semipronation, the right hip and knee in extreme flexion, and the left hip and knee in slight flexion. The knee-chest or proctoscopic position is also acceptable, but only if the rectal examination is to be followed with a proctosigmoidoscopy. The position permitting the most complete rectal examination is one with the patient lying supine, the knees flexed, and, if possible, the pelvis elevated on a pillow. One hand passes between the legs and explores the rectum while the other hand palpates the patient's abdomen. This position sometimes makes it possible to palpate tumors that otherwise would not be discovered on rectal examination.

The perineum

Inspection of the perineum may give important information. Fistulae, hemorrhoids, condylomas, dermatitis, swellings, ulcers, or prolapse may be seen. Finding fistulae in a patient with chronic diarrhea should lead you to suspect Crohn's disease of the small or large intestine.

Rectal examination should be preceded by palpation of the perianal region. This may reveal fistulous tracts, which are felt like cords oriented toward the anus.

Rectal palpation

Rectal palpation should be done carefully; otherwise, important lesions may be overlooked. Introduce a well-lubricated, gloved finger slowly and gently, with the transverse diameter parallel to the anterior-posterior axis of the anus. Once the finger is fully in the rectum, the inexperienced physician may be content with alternately flexing and extending the two distal phalanges and, not feeling anything abnormal, judge the examination to be negative. Except in the case of foreign bodies, pathology of the rectum involves its walls. These should be methodically palpated. The following method is recommended: First feel the posterior wall, identifying the levator and piriform muscles at the upper posterolateral area, and the mobility and sensitivity of the coccyx. Then, anteriorly, check the prostate in men and the uterine cervix in women. From here, slip the finger over all the rectal mucosa, checking for masses. If you find any, determine their exact location and whether they are covered with mucosa. Finally, ask the patient to bear down as if he were defecating and palpate for tumors.

A common error of beginners is to omit methodical palpation of the walls of the rectum. Another common mistake is to confuse the uterine cervix with an intrarectal tumor. It's so easy to do this that it's wise to identify the cervix *before* exploring for abnormalities.

On entering the rectum, the examining finger may, without recognizing it, push up a tumor. It is therefore better to introduce the finger as far as possible without touching the walls, then bend it slightly and pull back, meanwhile feeling the rectal walls. This procedure should be repeated along each one of the cardinal points. This increases the chances of finding a tumor or other lesion that displaces the wall.

On withdrawing it, always wipe the gloved finger with gauze and examine the secretion or fecal matter that adheres to it. This is an excellent opportunity to examine the adhering fecal matter for occult blood by means of the guaiac test.

Ninety per cent of carcinomas of the rectum can be felt on rectal examination. When they are small, they are low and flat, or nodular with an indurated base. When the center is ulcerated, you can feel a superficial depression with indurated base and raised, everted border. Whenever you find this, determine its proximal end, its size, whether its form is anular, tubular, ulcerated, or cauliflower-like, its fixation to surrounding structures, and its distance from the anus.

Adenomatous polyps are felt as pedunculated or sessile tumors, sometimes slightly lobulated and firm. In contrast, villous adenomas are soft and velvety, sometimes gelatinous; like malignant tumors, they bleed easily.

Inspection of the stool

This examination must under no circumstances be overlooked. Chapter 12 details possible findings and their diagnostic significance.

Bibliography

Bartholomew LG, Cain JC, Perry HO, et al: Cutaneous manifestations of gastrointestinal disease. *Postgrad Med* 36:247, 1964

Masters R, Herskovic T: Cutaneous manifestations of disorders of the alimentary tract. In *Dermatology in General Practice,* pp 1347–1349. New York: McGraw-Hill, 1971

Reid JD: Intestinal carcinoma in the Peutz-Jeghers syndrome. *JAMA* 229:833, 1974

Winawer SJ, Sherlock P, Shatterfeld D, et al: Screening for colon cancer. *Gastroenterology* 70:783, 1976

Wormsley KG: *The Skin and Gut in Disease.* London: Pitman, 1964

Chapters 12 and 13 are summarized in Chapter 14.

Summary of clinical diagnosis

14

As in so many medical problems, a careful, complete history and physical examination give the basic information in regard to etiology of diarrhea. At this point, you may suspect:

☐ The physiopathology causing the diarrhea
☐ The segment(s) of the gastrointestinal tract or other organs most likely involved in the diarrheal disease
☐ The probable cause(s).

Examples:
Characteristics of a dysenteric syndrome:

1. The stools consist basically of mucopurulent exudate
2. The affected areas are the rectum and distal colon

3. The probable causes are invasive amebiasis, non-specific ulcerative colitis, infection with enteric bacteria, or tumors; tumors can be felt in many cases on rectal examination.

Characteristics of a colitic syndrome:

1. The colon is the segment involved
2. Psychic disturbances or inflammatory lesions or tumors are the cause.

The pathophysiology of diarrhea in colitis is not always easy to determine. In many cases, abnormal motility of the colon is part of the picture. In most underdeveloped countries, colitis is the most common cause of chronic diarrhea and in the vast majority of cases the etiology is inflammatory (amebas and other parasites). Lactase deficiency, however, is more common than was originally suspected. The irritable bowel syndrome is also very common, particularly in urban areas. In developed countries, nonspecific chronic inflammatory bowel disease is probably the leading cause of chronic diarrhea. Signs and symptoms localizing the process to the small intestine are difficult to differentiate from those pointing to the colon as the site of pathology.

The typical malabsorption syndrome has such definitive signs and symptoms that it's easy to diagnose. In many cases, its etiology can be suspected: celiac disease in children, which is the same as gluten enteropathy in adults; tropical sprue when clinical findings, epidemiology, and geographic data support the diagnosis; surgery (iatrogenic); systemic sclerosis; and Whipple's disease. Of all these, celiac disease in children and gluten enteropathy are seen most frequently. On clinical grounds, you may suspect such conditions as intolerance to milk, intolerance to disaccharides, bacterial overgrowth, insufficiency of bile salts, pancreatic diarrhea, or gastrogenic diarrhea.

Diarrheas of extradigestive origin are not difficult to diagnose if you keep them in mind. Emotional tension and the various endocrinopathies should be systematically ruled out in all patients with chronic diarrhea.

It's evident that you can arrive at a correct diagnosis in the great majority of cases on the basis of clinical data alone.

You can then direct further study along really important lines, and omit superfluous examinations, which are often costly and bothersome. Some studies, however, should never be omitted: proctosigmoidoscopy, examination of the stool for bacteria and parasites, chemical and microscopic stool examination, and a barium enema. These are routine examinations and should be done on all patients with chronic diarrhea. Colonoscopy is rightly becoming another important diagnostic and therapeutic procedure, but its abuse should be avoided.

Proctosigmoido-scopic examination

15

Proctosigmoidoscopy should be done in all cases of chronic diarrhea. It establishes the diagnosis in the following conditions:

☐ Anorectal diseases such as hemorrhoids, condylomas, cryptitis and papillitis, ulcers, and anal fistulae, which are not necessarily related to the diarrhea

☐ Proctitis and colitis due to amebae, nonspecific ulcerative colitis, pseudomembranous enterocolitis, candidiasis, lymphogranuloma venereum, tuberculosis, ischemic and radiation proctitis and colitis

☐ Benign tumors: simple and adenomatous, villous adenomas, multiple familial polyposis

☐ Malignant tumors: adenocarcinoma.

Appendix A describes proctosigmoidoscopic technique and briefly compares the types of instruments.

Amebic proctitis and colitis

Most cases of amebic proctitis and colitis present a typical endoscopic picture: ulcers of different sizes, round or oval, covered with a whitish membrane that reveals a bleeding surface when removed. These ulcers may vary from early, superficial lesions measuring only a few millimeters in diameter to large, deep craters with jagged edges containing necrotic areas and mucous membrane tags that look like pseudopolyps. The intestinal wall between these ulcers appears to be normal except in very severe cases. The exudate from these ulcers contains vegetative forms of *Entamoeba histolytica,* which may be seen easily if the secretion is examined immediately, while it is still warm, under the microscope.

The diagnosis of nonspecific ulcerative colitis is made by proctosigmoidoscopy since the mucosa of the rectum and sigmoid colon is involved in the vast majority of cases. In the early stages, the changes in the mucosa are minimal, making diagnosis difficult. Numerous petechiae just under the epithelium give the mucosa a mottled appearance. The mucous membrane is friable and bleeds easily when rubbed with a cotton swab or with the sigmoidoscope.

In advanced stages, the changes in the mucosa are more pronounced and point more clearly to the diagnosis. The mucous membrane is frankly congested, edematous, and granular. Large amounts of mucus are secreted and there is bleeding on the slightest contact. In this stage, small, superficial ulcers may occur, especially in the distal segment of the rectum.

In more advanced stages, bleeding and ulceration are even more evident. Copious bleeding of the mucosa may interfere with the endoscopic examination. The ulcerated areas may be extensive, covered with blood and thick, mucopurulent exudate, and separated by areas of red, edematous, granular mucosa.

In fulminating cases, the sigmoidoscope should be introduced with extreme caution because of the fragility of the co-

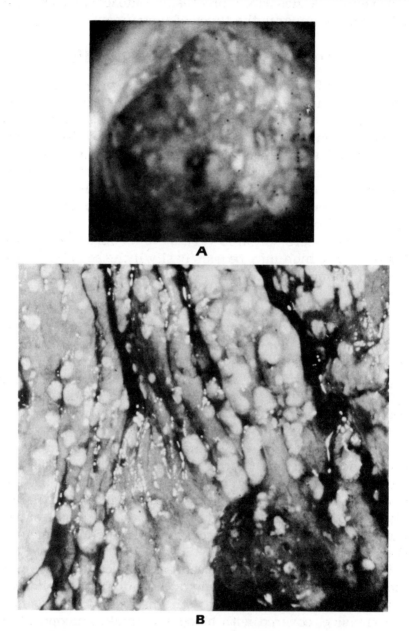

FIGURE 15-1 **Pseudomembranous enterocolitis**
A. Sigmoidoscopic appearance   B. Postmortem

lonic walls. It will show large ulcerated areas covered with bloody, mucopurulent exudate, surrounded by swollen, irregular, granular, gelatinous mucosa.

When the condition is chronic, the sigmoidoscopic pictures during exacerbation and remission are different. During an exacerbation, the intestine is narrowed, tubular, and stenotic in places; the mucosa is gelatinous, edematous, and bloody with some areas of polypoid hyperplasia and others completely denuded. During remission, the tubular appearance and stenotic zones persist. There is no peristalsis and the sigmoidoscope passes easily, almost by gravity. The mucosa, instead of being congested and swollen, is pale, nonfragile, and free of exudate. Pseudopolyps may be seen. They differ from true adenomatous polyps by being softer and incompletely covered with epithelium. They are witness to the regenerative capacity of the intestinal mucous membrane.

Pseudomembranous enterocolitis

This condition is seen in patients who have taken broad-spectrum antibiotics, who have had surgery, usually abdominal, or who are suffering from debilitating diseases. It's characterized by diarrhea and fever. The stools are liquid and contain mucus, pus, and sometimes blood. They are very abundant, often causing severe dehydration, electrolyte imbalance, shock, and death. Smears from the stools may show abundant *Staphylococcus aureus,* coagulase-positive. Sigmoidoscopy is essential for the diagnosis. It shows a congested, fragile mucosa, dotted with yellowish-white plaques that cover an erythematous base. Sometimes the plaques become confluent, forming false membranes from which the name of this syndrome is derived (Figure 15-1) (see Chapter 34).

Candidial colitis

Colitis due to overgrowth of *Candida* is becoming more common because of the use and abuse of broad-spectrum antibiotics, which destroy the ecologic balance of the colon and favor the excessive growth of molds and yeasts. The endoscopic picture is nonspecific. The mucosa is inflamed and often there is mucus and bloody exudate. The diagnosis is made on the basis of a recent history of taking antibiotics, pruritus ani, often vaginal candidiasis, and many yeast organisms in the stools.

Granulomatous colitis

In granulomatous colitis, or Crohn's disease of the colon, the rectum is usually spared. This is an important diagnostic point in differentiating it from nonspecific ulcerative colitis. If the rectosigmoid segment is involved, the mucosa is edematous, with elevations that give it a cobblestone appearance, and small, isolated ulcers are seen. In mild cases there is no fragility and no diffuse granulation, so characteristic of nonspecific ulcerative colitis. Instead, there are focal areas of edema and petechiae separated by areas of normal mucosa. In other cases, there are small ulcers resembling amebic ulcers. The latter can be diagnosed only by finding the vegetative forms of *Entamoeba histolytica* in the exudate or in a biopsy of the lesion.

Tuberculous proctocolitis

This complication of pulmonary tuberculosis is rarely seen because effective treatment is available for the primary disease. Endoscopic examination shows an inflamed mucosa dotted with ragged, elliptical ulcers whose long axes are placed transversely. Bacterial examination of the exudate may help in establishing the diagnosis.

Benign tumors

Benign tumors of the rectum and sigmoid do not cause diarrhea unless they are very large or numerous or secrete great quantities of liquid mucus. Diagnosis by sigmoidoscopy is easy. Sometimes these tumors appear as tiny hemispherical elevations, a few millimeters thick, and barely visible since their surface is so similar to the surrounding mucous membrane. Larger tumors may have an embossed and sometimes ulcerated surface. If they are pedunculated, they may have a long or short, thin or thick pedicle.

Adenoma

Villous or papillary adenoma is of interest because of its malignant potential and because it secretes copious amounts of mucus rich in electrolytes. It causes diarrhea and can be responsible for important loss of water, sodium, and potassium. These sessile tumors are joined to the mucosa of the rectum by a large, wide base. They are recognized by their many delicate epithelial fronds, their softness (making palpation difficult), and their great fragility. The free edge of the sigmoidoscope easily breaks off fragments of the tumor.

Multiple familial polyposis

The sigmoidoscopic appearance of multiple familial polyposis is pathognomonic. The mucous membrane is covered with so many small sessile polyps of uniform size that areas of normal mucous membrane are scarce. Only the beginner would confuse them with the extensive pseudopolyposis of nonspecific ulcerative colitis. In nonspecific ulcerative colitis, pleomorphism, ulceration, and fragility make the differential diagnosis easy.

Carcinoma

Carcinoma of the sigmoid and rectum can be diagnosed by proctosigmoidoscopy. The tumor varies in form. It may be nodular, scirrhous, colloid, or papillary. Nodular tumors project into the intestinal lumen as irregular, sessile, ulcerated masses. Scirrhous tumors, however, cause progressive narrowing of the lumen with hardening and infiltration of the intestinal walls. Mucinous or colloid adenocarcinoma is soft and gelatinous and bleeds easily at the slightest contact. Papillary adenocarcinoma looks like the villous adenoma from which it arises and is characterized by its wide base, softness, friability, and long, delicate fronds.

TABLE 15-1

Causes of chronic diarrhea
that can be diagnosed following clinical
and proctosigmoidoscopic study

Nonspecific ulcerative colitis
Polyps of the rectum and sigmoid
Villous adenoma of the rectum and sigmoid
Carcinoma of the rectum and sigmoid
Iatrogenic diseases of the intestine
Radiation enteritis and proctitis

TABLE 15-2

Causes of chronic diarrhea that may be
strongly suspected following
clinical and proctosigmoidoscopic study

Irritable colon
Ulcerative proctocolitis
  Nonspecific
  Granulomatous
  Amebic
  Tuberculous
Pseudomembranous enterocolitis
Regional enteritis
Intestinal tuberculosis
Lactose intolerance
Malabsorption syndrome
  Celiac sprue
  Tropical sprue
  Abnormal bacterial overgrowth
  Gastrointestinal surgery

Scleroderma
Ischemia
Carcinoid
Pancreatic insufficiency
Liver disease
Biliary tract disease
Hyperthyroidism
Adrenal insufficiency
Diabetes mellitus (autonomous
  neuropathy)

Ischemic colitis

Findings in ischemic colitis are nonspecific: multiple small ulcers and polypoid or nodular lesions that may be colored blue-black by the underlying blood. Findings on rectal biopsy are likewise nonspecific, but in some cases frank ischemic necrosis is seen.

Radiation enteritis and proctitis

This is seen especially in women who have had irradiation for cervicouterine cancer. The rectal mucosa is fragile, friable, and granular with multiple telangiectases. These are typical and predominate on the periphery of necrotic and ulcerated areas. Stenosis often occurs above the ulcerated area, 10 to 12 cm from the anus.

Colitis cystica profunda

This is a rare cause of diarrhea. It's characterized by the formation of cysts full of mucus under the muscularis mucosae of the distal colon. Patients complain of diarrhea, tenesmus, and discharge of mucus, which because of its high potassium content may cause important loss of this electrolyte. Rectal palpation reveals soft, movable masses, which through the sigmoidoscope look like polyps covered with normal mucosa. Sometimes the mucosa appears not unlike that in colitis, leading some authors to believe that this is an inflammatory process. Large lesions should be removed surgically.

SUMMARY

After taking a complete clinical and personal history, making a rectal examination, inspecting the feces, and doing a proctosigmoidoscopic study, you can determine whether the patient has one of the diarrheal diseases listed in Tables 15-1 and 15-2. Those listed in Table 15-2 require further tests for documentation and confirmation.

Routine laboratory examination of stools

16

A careful examination of the feces is essential for any patient suffering from diarrhea. A stool culture and a search for ova and cysts in three fecal samples are the minimum requirements. Thanks to this procedure it's possible to identify a high percentage of the bacteria, protozoa, and helminths that are responsible for causing diarrhea: bacteria of the Enterobacteriaciae family such as *Shigella; Salmonella* and pathogenic strains of *Escherichia coli;* the protozoans *Entamoeba histolytica, Giardia lamblia, Balantidium coli;* and helminths such as *Ascaris lumbricoides, Enterobius vermicularis, Necator americanus, Ancylostoma duodenale, Trichuris trichiura, Strongyloides stercoralis, Taenia* saginata, T. solium, Diphyllobothrium latum, and *Hymeno-lepis nana.* In some cases it might be necessary to perform additional special studies, such as smears for *Staphylococcus aureus* and *Candida* in patients suffering from antibiotic-related diarrhea, or cultures of anaerobes in intestinal fluids obtained through aspiration in patients with bacterial overgrowth syndromes.

Besides the bacteriologic and parasitologic information obtained by the stool examination, other important clues may be obtained, such as the presence of excessive amounts of fat or large numbers of leukocytes.

For stool cultures the samples must be fresh. The patient should defecate in the laboratory unless he is hospitalized or the fecal sample can be taken directly during proctoscopic examination. In some laboratories the sample is taken directly from the rectum, using cotton swabs or a glass spoon lubricated with nutrient broth. It's likewise important to place the material in culture medium as soon as possible. If this must be delayed more than one or two hours, the sample should be refrigerated.

Negative stool cultures do not rule out pathogenic organisms. Elimination of these bacteria in the feces is intermittent and irregular. As a result, about 30 per cent cannot be diagnosed from laboratory studies.

If the culture is positive, the next step is to test for sensitivity to various antibiotics. This is important because many bacteria have become resistant to antibiotics that were effective in the past.

In looking for parasites, if the patient is currently having diarrhea, *fresh* specimens should be examined immediately in order to find the vegetative forms of the protozoa. Otherwise, cysts and eggs can be looked for in solid stools using the concentration technique and examining three or more stools in sequence.

After this, a saline laxative should be given, and the resulting stools examined immediately. This step is left to the last because the effect of the laxative markedly decreases the concentration of cysts and eggs in the stool for several days. The chances of finding amebic trophozoites is increased immediately following administration of a laxative because the cecum, a favorite spot for invasive amebiasis, is emptied by the laxative's action.

A saline laxative, not castor oil, should be used. Drops of oil interfere with microscopic examination. Nor should the stool be mixed with urine or barium. Urine destroys the vegetative forms of the protozoa, and barium makes the examination impossible.

Many parasitologists recommend examining stools every two or three days to increase the chances of finding cysts, since they are not expelled daily. Solid stools should be collected in clean glass or waxed cardboard containers. Nothing should be added—no detergents or disinfectants of any kind. The stools should be examined soon after they're passed. If that is not possible, they should be refrigerated to preserve the cysts and eggs of parasites. This is not true of the vegetative forms, which die rapidly on cooling.

You can use the proctoscope to obtain samples of fecal matter and other material directly from the lesions of the mucosa. A pipette for aspirating material or a spoon for scraping the lesions is preferable to a cotton swab. It may be best to take a biopsy and look for parasites in the histologic sections.

Make sure that the parasitologist or laboratory technician who does the work is competent. The identification of eggs and cysts, especially cysts and vegetative forms of *Entamoeba histolytica,* is not always easy. These are often confused with nonpathogenic protozoa and with cells and other material in the stools.

The finding of pathogenic bacteria, protozoa, or helminths should not automatically establish a cause-and-effect relationship with the diarrhea. These parasites may cause spells of acute diarrhea but they are not responsible for chronic diarrhea. The two exceptions are giardiasis and invasive amebiasis. Giardiasis can cause chronic diarrhea and malabsorption syndrome (Chapter 31). Amebiasis is more likely to produce intermittent diarrhea but sometimes may cause dysentery and colitis that last for weeks or even months (Chapter 30).

In a patient with acute diarrhea, finding intestinal parasites suggests a causal relationship. which may be checked by observing the effect of treatment. In chronic diarrhea, however, finding parasites may prove only their concomitant existence in a person who is a carrier. This is particularly important regarding the diagnosis of amebiasis. Finding cysts of *E. histolytica* does not make a diagnosis of invasive amebiasis. Often this is a commensal form of the parasite that does not have invasive properties. Many patients with chronic diarrhea are treated time and again with all kinds if antiamebic drugs with little or no results. These patients may come to suffer from a real "amebic paranoia," and quite a number of physicians seem to be victims of the same ailment.

It's possible, on the other hand, for the most careful search to fail to reveal bacteria, protozoa, or other pathogenic elements that are actually present. This happens in one-third of cases of acute infections with enteric bacteria. It also happens in 50 per cent of cases of giardiasis and in an unknown number, undoubtedly high, of amebiasis. Fortunately, duodenal aspiration and peroral biopsy of the small intestine in the case of giardiasis are valuable diagnostic techniques. They are reviewed in Appendices C and B, respectively. Likewise, hemagglutination reactions in invasive amebiasis are most helpful. These complementary procedures are of enormous importance since giardiasis and amebiasis are such frequent causes of human diarrhea.

Bibliography

Blair JE, Lennette EH, Truant JP: *Manual of Clinical Microbiology.* Bethesda, Md: American Society for Microbiology, 1970

Harris JC, DuPont HL, and Hornick RB: Fecal leukocytes in diarrheal illness. *Ann Intern Med* 76:697, 1972

Olarte J: Diagnostico bacteriologico de las diarreas. In *Enfermedades Diarreicas en el Nino,* p 67. Mexico: Ediciones Medicas Hospital Infantil, 1973

Sawitz WG, Faust EC: The probability of detecting intestinal protozoa by successive stool examinations. *Am J Trop Med Hyg* 22:131, 1972

SUMMARY

A stool culture and search for ova and cysts in three fecal samples are mandatory. In the majority of cases they lead to identification of bacteria, protozoa, and helminths as causative agents. At times smears for *Staphylococcus* and *Candida* or aspirated intestinal fluid cultures for anaerobes may be necessary. Other characteristics of the stool, such as excessive fat or large numbers of white cells, also give important information. Samples should be as fresh as possible. If the bacterial culture is positive, antibiotic sensitivity tests are in order. A saline laxative after a diarrheal fresh specimen will empty the cecum, a favorite spot for invasive amebiasis. It will often expose the organism. Organisms discovered in this way are often the cause of acute diarrhea but not of the chronic variety, except for *Giardia lamblia* and invasive *Entamoeba histolytica.* Frequently amebae are found in carriers and are not related to the prevailing diarrhea. Where no organism is found in this way, duodenal aspiration and peroral small intestine biopsy may secure the diagnosis, especially of giardiasis. Hemagglutination reactions can be helpful in the diagnosis of invasive amebiasis.

Serology in amebiasis

17

In 1968 the first axenic—bacteria-free—culture was made of *Entamoeba histolytica*. It opened the way to making pure parasitic antigens. Thus amebic serology was born and various reactions developed for diagnostic purposes. The most significant is the indirect hemagglutination reaction. Both sensitive and specific, it's positive in 98 per cent of amebic liver abscesses and in more than 80 per cent of cases of invasive amebiasis of the colon. On the other hand, it's negative in 98 per cent of patients with no evidence of amebiasis and in 95 per cent of asymptomatic carriers of *E. histolytica*. Other tests currently employed for detecting this parasite are indirect immunofluorescence, contraimmune electrophoresis, and agar gel diffusion; all of these laboratory techniques produce essentially the same results.

The indirect hemagglutination test is considered positive when the titer is 1 : 128 or more. Remember that the agglutination titer is not proportional to the extent of tissue invasion, but varies with individual factors. Also, the antibodies formed in response to the amebic invasion last for many years after the patient has been cured. Consequently, a positive reaction does not indicate an active infection; nor, if it is done following treatment, does it mean a therapeutic failure. The titers go down slowly over a long time. To date, there is no serologic test that differentiates between active infection and past or cured infection.

Serologic tests must be interpreted very cautiously when used for clinical diagnosis of amebiasis and weighed along with all the other clinical and laboratory data available in each case. The great value of these tests in epidemiologic studies needs no emphasis. A negative test in a patient thought to have extraintestinal or invasive intestinal amebiasis should lead to a critical re-examination of the evidence for the diagnosis.

An important application of serologic examination is in the screening of patients thought to have inflammatory bowel disease. Since no more than 2 per cent of these patients have positive antibody titers for *E. histolytica,* a positive test should raise the possibility that the patient has amebiasis. Because of the potentially fatal consequences of giving steroids to patients with amebic colitis and the uncertain quality of parasitologic stool examination in most U.S. laboratories, all those patients who are diagnosed as having inflammatory bowel disease should have a serologic test for amebiasis.

Bibliography

Healy SR: Laboratory diagnosis of amebiasis. *Bull NY Acad Med* 47:478, 1971

Healy SR, Kraft SC: The indirect hemagglutination test for amebiasis in patients with inflammatory bowel disease. *Am J Dig Dis* 17:97, 1972

Juniper K Jr: Parasitic diseases of the intestinal tract. In *Gastroenterologic Medicine* (Paulson M, ed), pp 472–555. Philadelphia: Lea & Febiger, 1969

Krogstad DJ, Spencer HC, Healy SR: Current concepts in parasitology. Amebiasis. *N Engl J Med* 298:262, 1978

SUMMARY

The most important serologic test for amebiasis is the indirect hemagglutination test. It is positive, at a titer of 1:128 or more, in 98 per cent of amebic liver abscesses and in more than 80 per cent of colonic invasion. It is negative in 98 per cent of those with no evidence of amebiasis and in 95 per cent of asymptomatic *E. histolytica* carriers. Because titers go down slowly, a positive reaction does not necessarily mean active infection. This test must be used as an adjunct to clinical signs and symptoms. All cases of "inflammatory bowel disease" should be screened with this test because of the potentially fatal use of steroids in amebic colitis.

Microscopic study of the stool in steatorrhea

18

In all cases of suspected steatorrhea, a microscopic examination for fat should be made. If the examination results in a positive finding, you can then order quantitative tests, which are much more difficult and costly. The microscopic examination, in contrast, is simple and can be done in any laboratory, no matter how small.

Normal stools contain few or no neutral fat globules. Be sure the patient has not taken an oil laxative such as mineral oil or castor oil! When many fat globules are found, it usually indicates steatorrhea due to deficiency of pancreatic enzymes. If the steatorrhea is due to malabsorption, staining the fecal matter with Sudan III does not reveal excess fat (unless acetic acid has been added). Although normal stools may contain large amounts of fatty acids, the globules are small. Up to 100 of these globules may be seen per microscopic field; their diameter varies from 1 to 4 μm. When an increase in fatty acids is mild, the globules are larger, from 1 to 8 μm. If 100 or more large globules are found in the field, this indicates mild steatorrhea.

In frank steatorrhea, all the fatty acid globules are large and there is hardly any fecal material around them. Finding more than 100 large globules, from 6 to as much as 75 μm in diameter, per microscopic field indicates a definite increase in fecal fat.

The technique is as follows: Place a small sample of stool, about 0.5 cm in diameter, on each of two slides. Examine the first one for neutral fats. Add two drops of water and thoroughly mix it with the feces. Then thoroughly mix in two drops of 95 per cent ethyl alcohol. Add two drops of Sudan III dye in 95 per cent ethyl alcohol. Mix this in with the edge of the coverslip and then cover the slide immediately. Under the high dry objective with 430 d magnification, examine the specimen for fat globules. They will be seen as yellow or orange refractile globules that tend to gather at the edges of the coverslip.

In the second slide, look for products of fat digestion. To accomplish digestion, add several drops of 36 per cent acetic acid to separate the soaps and other fatty acids, followed by several drops of Sudan III. Mix this preparation, cover it with a coverslip, and gently heat it over an alcohol lamp until it begins to boil. Repeat this procedure rapidly two or three times to melt the fatty acid crystals. Examine the preparation while it is still hot, via the high dry objective with magnification of 430 d. The stained fatty acids will appear as dark orange globules while still hot, and they will crystallize on cooling.

Bibliography

Drummey GD, Benson JA Jr, Jones CM: Microscopical examination of the stool for steatorrhea. *N Engl J Med* 264:85, 1961

SUMMARY

Normal stools contain few or no fat globules. Where many are found, it usually means steatorrhea due to pancreatic enzyme deficiency. Malabsorption may produce steatorrhea. One hundred or more fat globules 1 to 8 μm in diameter per microscopic field represent mild steatorrhea; more than 100 large globules 6 to 75 μm indicate a definite increase in fecal fat.

Tests for lactose intolerance

19

An important advance in modern medicine was the discovery that lactase deficiency is common in adults and that frequently this deficiency causes diarrhea and other symptoms that can be confused with irritable colon (see Chapters 5 and 39). When these individuals ingest milk or milk products in excess of their lactase supply the symptoms appear. All patients with chronic diarrhea, whose history suggests lactose intolerance, should have a lactose tolerance test.

The test is done as follows: Lactose dissolved in water is given orally. Amounts vary. Some workers use a total of 50 gm, or 50 gm/square meter of surface area in children, dissolved in 250 to 500 ml of water. The patient is observed for

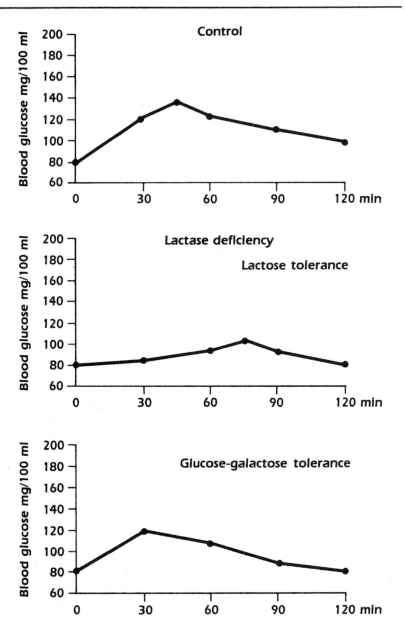

FIGURE 19-1   **Absorption of lactose and glucose-galactose in a
healthy person (top) and a patient with lactase deficiency (center, bottom)**

the next six hours and diarrhea, abdominal pain, or borborygmi are noted. Blood samples, preferably capillary blood, are taken at intervals of 0, 15, 30, 60, 90, and 120 minutes following the ingestion of lactose, and the total reducing matter in the blood is determined by the ferrocyanide test. Glucose may be determined by the glucose oxidase technique. If the curves are flat, it is important to follow this up with a tolerance test of the two monosaccharides making up the disaccharide being studied (galactose and glucose in the case of lactose) in equimolar amounts totaling the same number of grams as the original disaccharide and to compare the results of the two tests (Figure 19-1).

In lactase deficiency, the rise in blood glucose is less than 25 mg/100 ml. The diagnostic value of the lactose tolerance test is controversial. Up to 30 per cent of subjects with normal lactase activity, as proven by small intestinal biopsy, may show a flat curve. Some authors have taken the view that the test is of no value and should be discarded. It is true that variations in gastric emptying and the use of venous blood may be sources of error. These can be avoided by giving lactose by tube directly into the duodenum and by measuring the glucose levels in capillary rather than venous blood. A practical approach, suggested by Bayless, is the following:

1. Do not test diabetic patients, who would be likely to show high blood glucose levels
2. If no symptoms occur and the glycemia rises more than 25 mg/100 ml, the diagnosis of lactase deficiency can be ruled out
3. If symptoms follow the ingestion of lactose but not of galactose and glucose and the peak of the glycemia is less than 25 mg/100 ml, there is lactase deficiency
4. If lactose produces symptoms but galactose and glucose do not and if the glycemic peak is over 25 mg/100 ml, it indicates lactose intolerance but not lactase deficiency; this is seen in 20 per cent of patients who do not tolerate milk
5. If lactose produces no symptoms and the glycemia peak is less than 25 mg/100 ml, probably this is not due to lactase deficiency but to a delay in gastric emptying.

The dose of lactose used in the test, 50 gm, is equal to the amount of lactose in a liter of milk. Ordinarily, a liter of milk is an excessive adult intake except in patients who are on a milk diet. A better test is to use 12 gm, which is the amount of lactose in a glass of milk. Studies on the lactose tolerance curves produced by testing with 12 gm are not available, but you can get a good idea as to the presence of lactase deficiency by observing for symptoms: abdominal pain, distention, flatulence, and diarrhea. Measuring the abdomen before and after the test determines the amount of distention. In children, the pH of the feces should be measured after giving lactose. If lactose is not digested and its components not absorbed, it undergoes bacterial fermentation in the colon, producing lactic acid, which makes the stools acid and lowers the pH. Two kinds of breath tests have been developed and are simpler than the standard lactose tolerance test: the CO_2 breath test and the hydrogen breath test. They are also more reliable (see Chapter 39).

Bibliography

Bayless TM, Rosensweig MS, Christopher N, et al: Milk intolerance and lactose tolerance tests. *Gastroenterology* 54:475, 1968

Donaldson RM Jr: Carbohydrate intolerance. In *Gastrointestinal Disease* (Sleisenger MH, Fordtran JS, eds), 2nd ed, vol 2, p 1181. Philadelphia: Saunders, 1978

Newcomer AD, McGill BD: Distribution of disaccharidase activity in the small bowel of normal and lactose deficient subjects. *Gastroenterology* 51:481, 1966

SUMMARY

All patients with chronic diarrhea whose history suggests lactose intolerance should have a lactose tolerance test. The ideal amount of lactose to be used is 12 gm dissolved in water. After swallowing this, the patient is observed for the next six hours for diarrhea, abdominal pain, and borborygmi. Blood is drawn at 0, 15, 30, 60, 90, and 120 minutes and the amount of reducing matter is determined by the ferrocyanide test and the glucose oxidase test. If the curves are flat, this should be followed by a galactose and glucose tolerance test, the two monosaccharides in equimolar amounts adding up to 12 gm of lactose. In lactase deficiency, the rise in blood glucose is less than 25 mg/100 ml. If lactose is not digested and absorbed, it undergoes putrefaction in the colon, producing lactic acid and lowering the pH of the stool.

X-ray studies

X-ray studies are unnecessary in acute diarrhea. In the chronic form they frequently give the clue to the diagnosis.

Four studies should be done routinely in patients with chronic diarrhea: chest X-ray, plain films of the abdomen, barium enema, and X-ray of the small intestine.

X-ray of the thorax

A chest X-ray in routine check-ups is customary. For patients with chronic diarrhea, this X-ray may reveal pertinent information in the following conditions:

□ Active pulmonary tuberculosis: this finding points to the possible existence of intestinal tuberculosis

- Amebic liver abscess: elevation and hypomobility of the right leaf of the diaphragm with a dome-shaped deformity, patches of atelectasis, pleural effusion, and even possible pulmonary abscess suggest liver amebiasis and, of course, intestinal involvement of the same etiology
- Bronchiectasis related to cystic fibrosis of the pancreas or to hypogammaglobulinemia: both these diseases may manifest themselves with diarrhea
- Metastases from neoplasms, possibly in the digestive tract: carcinoids, gastrinomas, carcinomas of the colon or rectum, etc.
- Pleural effusion in pancreatitis or from hypoproteinemia in protein-losing enteropathies.

Plain film of the abdomen

A careful study of plain films of the abdomen (Figure 20-1) can reveal much to the experienced and conscientious physician. In the case of a patient with chronic diarrhea, the following findings are important:

- Pancreatic calcifications: X-ray evidence of chronic pancreatitis and therefore suggestive of exocrine pancreatic insufficiency
- Gallstones: biliary insufficiency, a rare cause of chronic diarrhea; gallstones may be secondary to impaired absorption of bile acids because of a diseased ileum
- Hepatomegaly from amebiasis, cirrhosis, metastatic carcinoma, lymphoma, amyloidosis, all possible causes of diarrhea
- Splenomegaly from portal hypertension, lymphomas, amyloidosis
- Abnormal gas shadows: sentinel loop in the acute stage of chronic relapsing pancreatitis; dilated loops of small intestine in subocclusion, inflammation, malnourishment, or malabsorption syndrome; cystic pneumatosis complicating diseases that cause diarrhea, such as regional enteritis, ulcerative colitis, tu-

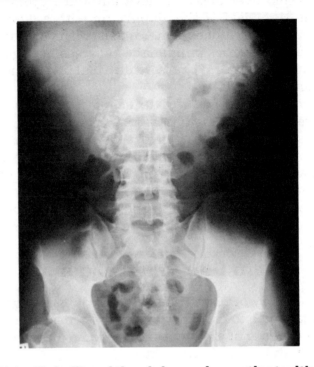

FIGURE 20-1   **Plain film of the abdomen in a patient with chronic pancreatitis**
Multiple pancreatic calcifications are evident. This patient had diabetes mellitus and steatorrhea

berculosis, lymphoma, or scleroderma of the small intestine

☐ Marked dilation of the large intestine, often confined to the transverse colon in toxic acute megacolon (Figure 20-2): a complication of nonspecific ulcerative colitis and also of invasive amebiasis of the colon. The transverse diameter of the dilated segment may reach 10 cm. The haustral markings disappear, the wall is thickened, and sometimes the gas penetrates into the intestinal wall through a deep ulcer. This causes a "double-contour" image with a translucent line running parallel to the principal gas shadow.

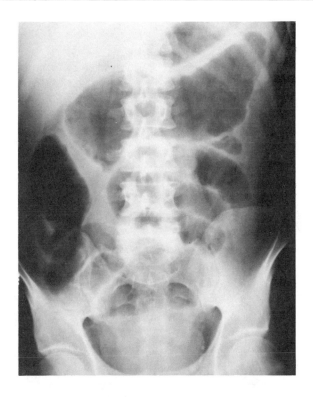

FIGURE 20-2 **Toxic megacolon in a patient with chronic ulcerative colitis**

X-ray of the colon

Adequate radiologic studies of the colon require a barium enema. This should be done in all patients with diarrhea if a definite diagnosis has not been made from previous studies. The barium is given by enema rather than by mouth because exact knowledge of pathologic changes of the colon, rather than its physiology, is the purpose of the study. A preliminary thorough cleansing of the colon with laxatives and/or enemas should be performed in order to identify swellings, ulcerations, diverticula, and mucosal changes, which are the anatomical substrata of many diarrheal diseases.

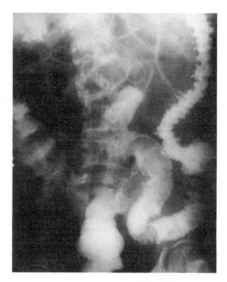

FIGURE 20-3 **Chronic ulcerative colitis**
Multiple ulcers are clearly apparent

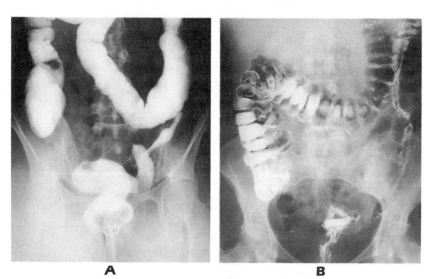

A B

FIGURE 20-4 **Long-standing chronic nonspecific ulcerative colitis**
A. The rectosigmoid has been shortened and narrowed until it is a rigid tube. B. Similar but more extensive changes

With the barium enema many inflammatory, neoplastic, and diverticular diseases of the colon can be diagnosed. The study may likewise be helpful in detecting functional derangements.

Nonspecific ulcerative colitis
Here, X-rays not only confirm the diagnosis suspected from clinical study and established by proctosigmoidoscopy but also give additional data of great value, such as the extent of the lesions, the degree of mucosal damage, and the presence of complications such as stenosis, pseudopolyps, carcinoma, perforations, and fistulae. However, X-rays are not infallible. In the early stages of the disease or when the process is localized to the rectum, the X-ray image may be entirely normal. Diagnosis of ulcerative proctitis is made by proctoscopy, not by X-rays.

Chronic nonspecific ulcerative colitis
In general, the X-ray changes are of three kinds: changes in the outline of the mucosa, disappearance or decrease of haustral markings, and narrowing and shortening of the involved segment.

The normal pattern of the mucosa is replaced by longitudinal folds, which result from epithelial destruction and hypertrophy. There are irregularities in the margins, which vary from a slightly raveled outline to a saw-toothed appearance with outgrowths of true ulcers (Figure 20-3), or a spotty picture caused by many pseudopolyps.

The loss of haustral markings is important if it shows up on every plate and if it coexists with shortening and narrowing of the colon and mucosal changes. Haustral markings may be diminished or absent in patients with irritable colon and in those who use too many laxatives. The latter do not show the other changes mentioned above.

Long-standing chronic nonspecific ulcerative colitis is characterized by a marked decrease in the caliber and length of the colon. It is not unusual to find it remarkably shortened and transformed into a rigid tube (Figure 20-4). At times the colon looks like a sausage because many areas of stenosis alternate with normal segments. The barium en-

TABLE 20-1

Radiologic differentiation between nonspecific chronic ulcerative colitis and granulomatous colitis

	Chronic ulcerative colitis	Granulomatous colitis
Distribution	Continuous, starting from the rectum	Discontinuous
Rectum	Almost always involved	Frequently normal
Anal fistulae	Occasional	Frequent
Internal fistulae	Absent	Possible
Stenosis	Absent	Frequent
Mucosa	Granular; superficial ulcers	Deep linear ulcers; cobblestone appearance
Small bowel	Normal or dilated; lesions are continuous with those in the proximal colon	Contracted, irregular; discontinuous lesions

ema allows the terminal ileum to be visualized, giving evidence as to its involvement with the disease.

Ileitis secondary to chronic nonspecific ulcerative colitis ("backwash ileitis") differs from Crohn's disease involving the terminal ileum. In Crohn's disease the involved segment is narrowed and becomes separated from the neighboring intestinal loops by inflammatory thickening of its walls; in ileitis secondary to chronic nonspecific ulcerative colitis, the image of the ileum is similar to that of the colon: dilated with rigidity and irregular borders.

Granulomatous colitis

Granulomatous colitis, or Crohn's disease of the colon, used to be confused with chronic nonspecific ulcerative colitis. Today it has its own identity. A set of radiologic, clinical, endoscopic, and histologic findings helps to establish the differential diagnosis. The differential X-ray findings are shown in Table 20-1. Figure 20-5 illustrates the radiologic characteristics of this disease.

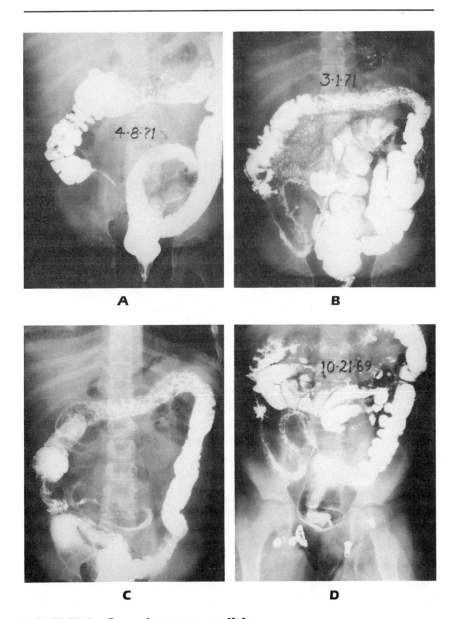

FIGURE 20-5 **Granulomatous colitis**
A. The distribution is discontinuous and the rectum has been spared.
B. There is an internal fistula. B and C. The mucosa has a cobblestone
appearance. B, C, and D. A Long segment of the ileum is involved.

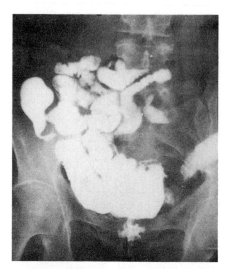

FIGURE 20-6 **Conical deformity of the cecum, characteristic of amebiasis**

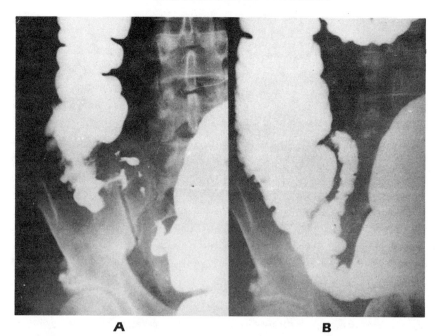

A   **B**

FIGURE 20-7 **Amebiasis of the cecum with typical conical deformity, before (A) and after (B) treatment**

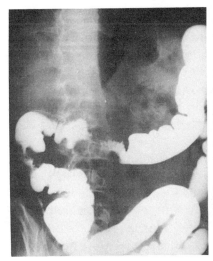

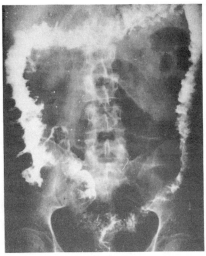

FIGURE 20-8 **Amebomas of the colon**

They resemble neoplastic filling defects

FIGURE 20-9 **Ulcerative amebiasis involving the entire length of the colon**

Invasive amebiasis of the colon

Here the radiologic abnormalities vary directly with the extent of colon involvement. When the disease is benign, the X-ray may be normal or may show mild irregularities in the contour of the diseased segment. If the process is more severe, the wall may be rigid. If the cecum is affected, the classic rigid conical deformity is produced (Figures 20-6 and 20-7). Ameboma is seen as thickening of the wall with localized narrowing of the colon either on one side of the wall or surrounding it. This picture is very difficult to differentiate from neoplasms and granulomatous colitis. Frequently, partial or complete healing of these lesions following treatment constitutes definite proof of the diagnosis (Figure 20-8). At times, amebiasis may involve the whole colon (Figure 20-9).

Intestinal tuberculosis

In intestinal tuberculosis the barium enema shows:

☐ Stierlin's sign: resistance to filling of the involved segment (cecum or terminal ileum) because of increased irritability; the barium is rapidly shunted into the adjoining segments, both proximal and distal

☐ Filling defects occur in the cecum similar to those seen in other granulomatous processes as well as in amebic and neoplastic lesions

☐ Fleischner's sign: the last 2 to 3 cm of the ileum form a triangle whose base faces the cecum, as a result of fibrosis of the lips of the ileocecal valve

☐ Shortening and deformity of the ascending colon

☐ Other changes in the small intestine, best seen by barium swallow but also visible by barium enema: obstructed, prestenotic, dilated areas with surrounding irregularities; prolonged retention of barium; thickening of folds; segmentation and stenosis of a whole segment, producing "string sign."

Diverticulosis of the colon

This common condition is probably asymptomatic. When there are symptoms, they are caused by concomitant conditions, such as an irritable colon. As diarrhea occurs in 20 to 45 per cent of these cases, however, it's well to review the X-ray picture briefly. The diverticula are small protrusions, round or pointed, with a diameter of 0.3 to 3 cm. Sometimes none or only a few are visible when the colon is full of barium, but after the barium has been expelled, many diverticula can be clearly seen. At times they are so numerous that the lumen of the colon is narrowed and the haustra are abolished. If irritable colon occurs along with diverticulosis, the outlines are irregular, or "irritable," and the lumen is twisted.

Polyps of the colon

Polyps of the colon do not cause diarrhea unless they are multiple or are villous adenomas (Chapter 37). Villous adenomas appear as localized filling defects on X-ray. They cannot be differentiated from adenomatous polyps or carcino-

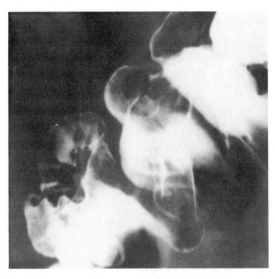

FIGURE 20-10 **Villous adenoma of the colon**

mas. Villous adenomas should be suspected when the adjacent wall is not infiltrated and when the filling defect has a spotty, lacy appearance changing in size and shape according to the amount of barium injected into the colon (Figure 20-10). Multiple polyposis is recognized radiographically by the many circular filling defects, best seen after the barium has been evacuated, or with double air contrast films (Figure 20-11). It's important to avoid confusing multiple polyposis with the pseudopolyposis of chronic ulcerative colitis, where, in addition to the filling defects in nonspecific ulcerative colitis, other characteristic changes are seen.

Carcinoma of the colon

Carcinoma of the colon can be diagnosed by X-ray or colonoscopy in nearly 100 per cent of cases. The X-ray findings are filling defects or localized areas of narrowing. These are usually abrupt and well circumscribed, and give the picture of a bitten apple core (Figure 20-12). The stenotic segment may be irregular and its morphology remains unchanged on every X-ray plate.

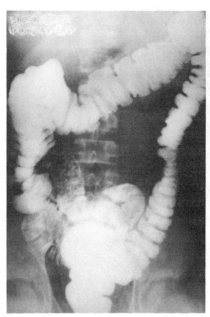

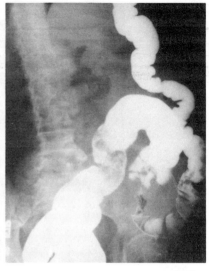

FIGURE 20-12 **Carcinoma of the sigmoid colon, visible as a narrowed, irregular, sharply demarcated area**
The patient had chronic diarrhea of three months' duration

FIGURE 20-11 **Multiple polyposis of the colon**

X-ray errors may arise from incomplete cleansing of the colon, leaving fecal masses that could be confused with a tumor or a polyp or could hide a tumor. Overlapping intestinal loops in the sigmoid colon and at the hepatic and splenic angles may result in poor visualization and can be avoided by proper technique.

The rectum is difficult to study by X-ray. Fortunately, it's accessible to palpation and visualization by proctoscopy. Proctosigmoidoscopy should always be done and should precede X-ray studies.

Irritable colon

The principal purpose of the barium enema in patients with irritable colon is to rule out organic lesions. Often other findings indicative of irritable colon are encountered: inordinate pain when the barium is introduced, difficulty in retaining it, spastic contractions, and exaggerated or absent haustra. The colon is not shortened as it is in nonspecific ulcerative colitis. For these findings to be significant, the colon must not have been traumatized by laxatives or irritating enemas and the barium must be introduced slowly and at body temperature.

X-ray of the small intestine

This is fundamental for the diagnosis of many illnesses accompanied by diarrhea. It is indispensable if up to this point the diagnosis has not been made.

Inspired by the masterly descriptions of Cherigié, Marshak, and their colleagues, we can classify the radiologic abnormalities of the small intestine caused by diarrhea-producing diseases into the following syndromes: functional syndrome, inflammatory syndrome, malabsorption syndrome, and other small intestinal diseases accompanied by diarrhea.

Functional syndrome

The functional syndrome shows several characteristic changes on X-ray.

Changes in motility. Hypomotility or hypermotility. In hypermotility, the barium may travel rapidly along the small intestine and arrive at the cecum in less than half an hour instead of taking the normal two to four hours.

Changes in tonicity. Hypertonia is usually accompanied by hyperperistalsis. The caliber is diminished, and the loops become thin and filiform and look like a rosary. These changes may be localized or extend throughout, giving the small intestine the appearance of "chicken gut."

Hypotonia is usually associated with hypoperistalsis. It is often seen in malabsorption syndromes. The loops are enlarged and girdled, with smooth borders. Gas and flocculation of the barium are often seen.

Retention of gas. The normal small intestine in the adult does not contain gas, since the normal mucosa absorbs it rapidly. Exceptions are cases of severe aerophagia, retrograde gas displacement through the ileocecal valve following enemas, and reflex dilation of small bowel loops in renal, pancreatic, bladder, or genital disease. Otherwise the presence of gas means an abnormal mucosa.

Retention of liquids. If there is no obstruction, retention of liquids in the intestine indicates interference with absorption or the presence of marked inflammation with or without hypersecretion. In such cases the barium appears dilute and flocculated.

Subocclusive syndrome. This is characterized clinically by colicky abdominal pain accompanied by visible and audible signs of hyperperistalsis terminating in the expulsion of gas and diarrheal stool. It is seen on X-ray as increased caliber of the intestinal loops, violent periodic peristaltic contractions attempting to pass a gas bubble, and, finally, passing it through a narrowed segment.

Occlusive syndrome. The basic X-ray finding is fluid and gas levels. The gas is seen as one or more bubbles above the fluid in the loop. The upper border of a single bubble is convex and regular, while its lower border is a horizontal line formed by the liquid level. When there are many bubbles, they are seen at varying levels, like stairsteps or organ pipes along an oblique axis that runs from the left hypochondrium to the right iliac fossa. Another finding is distended arcs also limited by fluid levels, especially in low obstruction. The walls are thin in mechanical obstruction, but in chronic disease and in inflammatory processes they are thickened by edema.

Inflammatory syndrome
Tuberculosis and regional enteritis are the two important inflammatory diseases of the small intestine that may cause chronic diarrhea. Their X-ray pictures are very similar. Often, however, the diagnosis cannot be made by X-ray but from other data such as the clinical picture, epidemiology, therapeutic tests, and biopsies.

Cherigié and colleagues divided the radiologically visible inflammatory changes of the intestine into functional and organic ones.

The functional derangements have been described: hyper- and hypomotility, hyper- and hypotonia, hyper- and hypoperistalsis, and retention of gas and fluids.

The organic changes may be divided into three stages: early, full-blown, and advanced. In the early stage, the X-ray shows mucosal edema and lymphoid hypertrophy. In the jejunum, mucosal edema causes thickening of the folds and slowing of the transit time. In the ileum, edema obscures the mucosal pattern and decreases intestinal flexibility, although not to the point of causing rigidity.

Lymphatic hypertrophy gives rise to the following:

☐ Enlargement of mesenteric lymph nodes, which, if excessive, may be seen as round, marginal, or central filling defects

☐ Hypertrophy of the lymphatic follicles that may appear polypoid, giving the loop a cobblestone or hobnailed appearance, especially in the terminal ileum

☐ Hypertrophy of Peyer's patches; normally invisible on X-rays, when hypertrophied they look like round or oval filling defects especially visible on the free border of the intestine.

In the full-blown stage, ulcerations of Peyer's patches or lymphatic follicles are the most important findings. Seen from the front, they look like roundish, opaque spots. From the side they appear as niches or spicules that stand out on the free border of the intestine. Usually they are multiple and separated from each other by areas that become rigid from edema surrounding the ulcers.

In the advanced stage, the intestine becomes fibrotic in the neighborhood of the ulcers, resulting in narrowing and segmental rigidity. Adhesions, perforations, and fistulae may bind the loops together. There are no pathognomonic X-ray changes that might differentiate intestinal tuberculosis from regional enteritis. However, the changes just described, common to both inflammatory enteropathies, have certain individual peculiarities.

Intestinal tuberculosis. At first, lymphoid hypertrophy is localized to the terminal ileum. Oval patches, giving a hobnailed appearance, or a large nodule on the free border of the intestine, which produces a true hollowed-out shadow ("alarm nodule" of Marina Fiol), may appear. Sometimes the bottom of the cecum is retracted. The tuberculous ulcers have irregular borders. Their long axis is usually transverse but may be longitudinal. Often the intestinal borders are spiny. Later the lesions extend to the cecum, whose base becomes dotted with radiolucent patches of hypertrophied lymphoid tissue. The borders become irregular because of small filling defects.

Functional changes consist of fragmentation of the barium column in the jejunum and ileum and hypertonicity of the terminal loop of the small intestine.

At the full-blown stage, the walls of the cecum become rectilinear and rigid, finally showing the classical Stierlin's sign: The cecal cavity does not fill and is reduced to a filiform tract. The small intestine shows spasmodic contractions and even stenosis. The functional signs are air bubbles, fluid levels, and dilated segments.

In the advanced stage, the lesions extend to the rest of the intestine and peritoneum. The loops coalesce and organic stenosis increases, causing subocclusion or a pseudo-tumoral hypertrophy that makes it difficult to differentiate from cancer. Cherigié has emphasized the great diagnostic value of a second area of disease involving a loop that appears suspended at the level of the right border of the fourth lumbar vertebra.

Regional enteritis (Crohn's disease). As in intestinal tuberculosis, early X-rays show hypertrophy of Peyer's patches. Later, the loop does not tolerate barium but contracts spasmodically and often becomes filiform with irregular outlines that bristle with spicules. As sclerosis progresses, the loop becomes more rigid (Figures 20-13 and 20-14).

In the full-blown stage, the terminal ileum and, less frequently, other segments of the small intestine and possibly of the colon are transformed into a narrow, rigid fibrotic

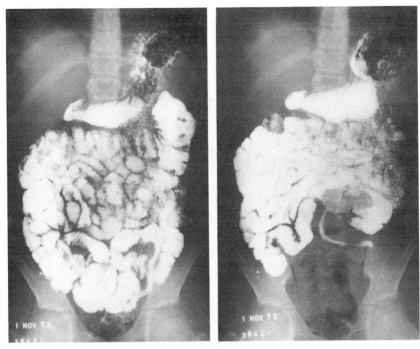

FIGURE 20-13 **Regional enteritis** FIGURE 20-14 **Regional enteritis**

passage that has been called the "string sign." Numerous spicules indicate the presence of ulcerations. The other intestinal loops are separated from the diseased one by a distance that corresponds to the marked thickening of the wall and the perivisceral inflammatory reaction. The segmental character of the lesion is shown by the sharp line of division between the diseased area and the adjoining healthy tissue.

In the advanced stages, the loops become clumped because of perivisceritis and mesenteritis. The disease may invade the ileocecal valve and cecum, creating lacunar areas that resemble tuberculosis, amebiasis, or neoplasms. In this advanced stage, fistulae form between loops. The fistulae are difficult to make out, but when they open into neighboring organs like the sigmoid or bladder, or onto the skin, they are easily visualized.

Malabsorption syndrome

Most diseases with deficient intestinal absorption show abnormalities of the small intestine called "nutritional deficiency pattern," "motor disturbance," or "segmentation pattern." These changes, which are especially marked in the advanced stages of celiac sprue, are termed the spruelike pattern.

The sprue pattern shows seven principal changes: dilation, segmentation, hypersecretion, thickening of the folds, changes in motility, moulage sign, and intussusceptions.

Dilation is one of the most important and constant X-ray findings in sprue. It is seen especially in the jejunum and varies greatly from one minute to the next during the examination, and from one patient to another. In general, its extent is related to the severity of the disease. The loops are long and winding with folded walls and prominent valves. Dilation seems to be due to intestinal hypotonia, permitting distention by foods and, perhaps, digestive juices.

Segmentation is also very common: Great masses of barium appear separate from each other in dilated loops full of secretions. This is seen especially in the ileum. Segmentation should not be confused with the scattering of the barium column (Figure 20-15), another finding in malabsorption syndrome, where remnants of the barium fragments look like soap flakes left straggling in the loops after most of the barium has been expelled.

Hypersecretion causes the barium to lose its normal homogeneous appearance and to look coarsely granular, with irregular areas of flocculation. The use of nonflocculating barium has made this sign less evident, since the diluted barium merely becomes less opaque.

The mucosal folds appear thickened, especially in the dilated loops. This is seen more clearly in some infiltrative or inflammatory diseases that give rise to the secondary malabsorption syndromes, especially lymphoma and Whipple's disease.

The velocity of intestinal transit varies in sprue. It's usually slowed to three to five hours or longer.

The moulage sign describes the X-ray picture of the jejunum in celiac sprue, where the folds are completely erased

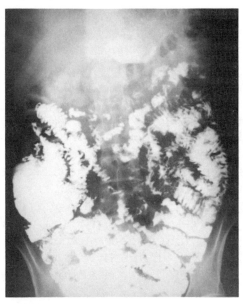

FIGURE 20-15 **Celiac sprue**
The barium is diluted and scattered from the presence of fluid, and the transit time is prolonged

and the barium-filled intestine looks like a solid wax mold.

Intestinal intussusceptions are seen frequently in sprue, and their presence supports the diagnosis. These processes do not obstruct the intestine and have a characteristic springlike appearance.

The combination of these seven findings suggests celiac sprue. They are nonspecific, however, and may be found in other diseases. Partial gastrectomy, steatorrhea from liver or bile duct disease, malnutrition, hookworm, and allergic or emotional diseases of the intestine may produce similar changes, though they may be less pronounced than in celiac sprue.

In diffuse lymphoma and Whipple's disease, the picture is also similar to that of sprue, but with more thickening of the folds. In lymphoma the increased thickening of the wall may suggest tumor infiltration.

Scleroderma of the small intestine causes dilation, sacculation, and marked hypomotility. Marked dilation of the second and third portions of the duodenum and characteristic changes in the esophagus help to establish the diagnosis.

Other diseases of the small intestine
Other diseases of the small intestine that occasionally cause diarrhea and can be diagnosed by X-ray include intestinal resections, short circuits, blind loops, dilated afferent loop, multiple diverticulosis, and some neoplasms such as lymphoma and, rarer still, carcinoid. The X-ray diagnosis is obvious in all of these except lymphoma and carcinoid tumor. X-ray diagnosis of carcinoid is particularly difficult, but occasionally a small filling defect associated with a sharp-angled bend in the small intestine, caused by retraction of the mesentery, is seen in this condition.

Bibliography

Boom RA, Garcia RH, Rios SG, et al: Signos radiologicos de la colitis amibiana fulminante. *Rev Gastroenterol Mex* 36:136, 1971

Cherigié E, Hillemand P, Proux C, et al: *L'Intestin Grêle Normal et Pathologique.* Paris: Expansion Scientifique Française, 1957

Marshak RH, Lindner AE: *Radiology of the Small Intestine,* 2nd ed. Philadelphia: Saunders, 1976

Wolf BS, Marshak RH: Granulomatous colitis (Crohn's disease of the colon): Roentgen features. *Am J Roentgenol* 88:662, 1962

SUMMARY

X-ray studies are unnecessary in acute diarrhea but may be of major significance in chronic diarrhea. Four studies are done routinely. Chest X-ray may reveal active pulmonary tuberculosis perhaps related to intestinal tuberculosis; amebic liver abscess; bronchiectasis possibly related to cystic fibrosis of the pancreas or hypogammaglobulinemia; metastases possibly from a gastrointestinal neoplasm; or pleural effusion due perhaps to pancreatitis or hypoproteinemia. A flat film of the abdomen may show pancreatic calcifications, gallstones, hepatomegaly, splenomegaly, abnormal gas shadows, or marked dilation of the large intestine. Barium enema (X-ray of the colon) will reveal chronic nonspecific ulcerative colitis, ileitis secondary to this, granulomatous colitis (Crohn's disease), invasive amebiasis of the colon at times with ameboma, diverticulosis of the colon, polyps, carcinoma, or irritable colon. X-ray of the small intestine will show the presence of functional syndrome, inflammatory syndrome, malabsorption syndrome, intestinal tuberculosis, regional enteritis (Crohn's disease), diffuse lymphoma, Whipple's disease, scleroderma, intestinal resections, short circuits, blind loops, dilated afferent loop, multiple diverticulosis, or carcinoid.

Colonoscopy

21

The most recent addition to the diagnostic armamentarium for patients with diarrhea is the colonoscope, or colonofibroscope. The best instrument now available is 1.86 meters long and can reach the cecum and reveal the ileocecal valve. It can be manipulated in four directions to show the entire circumference of the intestinal wall. It has an apparatus for insufflating the intestine with air and another for aspirating the intestinal contents. There is an opening for inserting sounds and swabs for taking samples, forceps for making biopsies, and hot wire loops for excising polyps. The apparatus is a semirigid tube with thousands of fine glass fibers that transmit light and images.

This equipment makes it possible to examine the whole colon and obtain definite information as to the location of hemorrhages in the lower bowel after the bleeding has stopped, polyps and multiple polyposis, villous adenomas, fistulae, carcinomas, amebomas, tuberculosis, nonspecific ulcerative colitis, and granulomatous and amebic colitis.

Compared with proctoscopy and X-rays colonoscopy is expensive, time-consuming, and not without risk. It should not be a substitute for these procedures of proved value but should supplement them when necessary. Colonoscopy with biopsy has been especially useful (1) when the barium enema shows abnormalities that cannot be exactly recognized, such as filling defects, narrowings, or polypoid images; (2) to determine the extent of an inflammatory process, since endoscopy is superior to X-ray; (3) when it is difficult to differentiate the different types of colitis; (4) to determine bleeding points in the lower intestine; and (5) to evaluate X-ray abnormalities in patients who have undergone surgery of the colon.

Colonoscopy is contraindicated in acute colitis, fulminating colitis, and toxic megacolon because of the danger of perforating the intestine. It is also contraindicated in suspected perforation of the colon, acute diverticulitis, and peritonitis.

Bibliography

Overholt BF: Colonoscopy. A review. *Gastroenterology* 68:1308, 1975

Schmitt MG Jr, Wu WC, Geenen JE, et al: Diagnostic colonoscopy. An assessment of the clinical indications. *Gastroenterology* 69:765, 1975

SUMMARY

The colonofibroscope, 1.86 meters long, can reach the cecum and reveal the ileocecal valve. The whole colon can be inspected with this instrument. It should be used only as a supplement to other procedures. It is especially useful when the barium enema shows unrecognizable defects, to determine the extent of an inflammatory process, to differentiate different types of colitis, to localize bleeding points in the lower intestine, and to evaluate X-ray findings in post-colonic-surgery patients. It is contraindicated in any acute colonic condition, including perforation and peritonitis.

Diagnosis and etiology of malabsorption syndrome

22

The great majority of the diseases causing chronic diarrhea can be diagnosed by X-ray and proctosigmoidoscopy—and when necessary by colonoscopy (Table 22-1). Among the diseases still awaiting diagnosis are those producing steatorrhea, the principal finding in the malabsorption syndrome. In typical malabsorption, the picture is so clear that it can be suspected clinically. Qualitative examination of the stool (Chapter 18) and X-ray of the small intestine give additional information that may establish the diagnosis. It's absolutely necessary in any case to proceed in an orderly fashion to arrive at the diagnosis and then to determine the condition's etiology.

TABLE 22-1

Diarrheal diseases that can be diagnosed after the laboratory and X-ray studies

---

Irritable colon
Colitis from parasites
Amebic ulcerative proctitis and colitis
Nonspecific ulcerative proctitis and colitis
Granulomatous colitis
Regional enteritis
Intestinal tuberculosis
Lactose intolerance
Scleroderma
Diarrhea secondary to gastric and intestinal surgery
Diabetic diarrhea

Clinical pictures

The patient with malabsorption syndrome may present three different pictures. (1) With the typical clinical picture, the diagnosis is easy and can be checked by appropriate laboratory studies. All that remains is to determine the etiology. (2) A patient who complains vaguely of dyspepsia, meteorism, flatulence, intermittent nonspecific pain, and diarrhea is often diagnosed as having irritable colon. The steatorrhea is subclinical and is discovered only on laboratory examination of the stool. The laboratory studies listed in Table 22-2 should be done on all patients with chronic diarrhea, dyspepsia, and flatulence. (3) When nutritional and metabolic changes have resulted from malabsorption, the digestive symptoms may be absent or not complained of by the patient, who will have various other symptoms, signs, and laboratory findings seen in Table 22-2.

Laboratory studies

Patients in any of these three groups should have the following studies: blood carotene, quantitative stool fats, D-xylose absorption, absorption of radioactive B_{12} or bile acid breath test, and biopsy of the small intestine.

Blood carotene

Low blood carotene is a strong indication of malabsorption syndrome. The test is relatively simple. It is not infallible, since 5 to 10 per cent of sprue patients have normal values, nor does it determine the origin of the malabsorption defect. Another source of error is a diet poor in carotene. To overcome this, the patient is instructed to take 50,000 units of vitamin A, or six carrots or three glasses of tomato juice daily, for three to five days prior to the test. With these precautions, the test is of great value, especially when it shows low carotene levels. If the blood carotene is low, the following studies are justified.

Quantitative test for stool fats

The clinical picture, qualitative study of stool fats, and blood carotene are useful in suspecting steatorrhea, a common finding in most malabsorption syndromes. But a definite diagnosis is made from the quantitative test for fat in the stools. If the patient takes 60 to 100 gm of fat daily for several days, omits any oily medication, has his usual number of bowel movements, and carefully collects all stools passed during a 72-hour period, more than 6 gm of fat excreted per day as measured by the modified Van de Kamer technique indicates steatorrhea.

For some time, studies of the absorption of triolein and oleic acid tagged with radioactive iodine were in vogue. It was thought that these studies would lead not only to a diagnosis of steatorrhea but to a differential diagnosis between steatorrhea of pancreatic and intestinal origin. It was believed that poor absorption of triolein from lack of lipase with normal absorption of oleic acid was an indication of pancreatic steatorrhea. Deficient absorption of both indicated intestinal steatorrhea. Unfortunately, results were not dependable and the test is not recommended. However, new tests based on ingestion of the fats tagged with ^{14}C, followed later by measurement of $^{14}CO_2$ in the expired air, show great promise.

TABLE 22-2

Symptoms, signs, and laboratory findings

Insufficient absorption of	Symptoms and signs	Laboratory findings
Water	Nocturnal diuresis	"Water test" abnormal
Electrolytes		
Sodium		Hyponatremia
Potassium	Polyuria	
	Abdominal distention	
	Ileus	Hypokalemia
	Tetany	Decreased total
	Asthenia	interchangeable
	Failure to gain weight	potassium
Calcium	Tetany	Hypocalcemia
	Bone pain	Osteomalacia
	Paresthesias	
Magnesium	Tetany	Hypomagnesemia
Vitamins		
A	Dry skin	Flat absorption curve of vitamin A
B	Glossitis, stomatitis, peripheral neuropathy	
D	Tetany	Hypocalcemia
	Bone pain	Hypophosphatemia
		Hypophosphatasemia
		Osteomalacia
K	Hemorrhages	Prolonged prothrombin time
B_{12}	Anemia	Decreased absorption of vitamin B_{12}
		Megaloblastic anemia

D-Xylose absorption test

D-Xylose is a five-carbon monosaccharide absorbed by passive and facilitated transport in the proximal part of the small intestine and eliminated in the urine. Apparently it is not metabolized by man but by bacteria, which normally do

in malabsorption syndrome

Insufficient absorption of	Symptoms and signs	Laboratory findings
Folic acid	Anemia	Megaloblastic anemia Flat absorption curve of folic acid
Iron	Anemia Koilonychia	Hypochromic anemia Decreased serum iron
Fats	Retarded growth Loss of weight Diarrhea Steatorrhea	Decrease in serum total lipids, phospholipids, cholesterol, carotene Increase in fecal fat Decrease in intestinal absorption of ^{131}I-labeled triolein and oleic acid
Carbohydrates	Retarded growth Weight loss Diarrhea Anal burning	Flat absorption curve of glucose, D-xylose, and disaccharides Decrease in fecal pH Lactosuria
Proteins	Retarded growth Weight loss Weakness Edema	Hypoproteinemia Increase in fecal nitrogen Marked increase in fecal protein Flat absorption curve of amino acids

not inhabit the proximal segments of the intestine. Twenty-five grams of D-xylose given orally to a fasting patient should result in the elimination of no less than 4.5 gm in the urine in the first five hours unless there is vomiting, severe hypothyroidism, slow gastric emptying, or renal insufficiency. Urinary excretion of less than 4.5 gm in five hours indicates a disturbance of jejunal function or bacterial overgrowth in the proximal intestine.

The D-xylose test is normal in some kinds of steatorrhea—i.e., exocrine pancreatic insufficiency, biliary insufficiency not caused by bacterial overgrowth, intestinal lymphomas, abetalipoproteinemia, and diseases or previous resection of the ileum. It is abnormal in all other malabsorption syndromes, especially celiac sprue, tropical sprue, abnormal bacterial overgrowth, extensive resections of the small intestine or the jejunum, gastrocolic fistulae, and gastroileal anastomosis.

B_{12} absorption test

This test of the absorptive capacity of the distal small intestine parallels the D-xylose test, which measures the same function in the proximal part. In addition, like D-xylose, vitamin B_{12} serves as a metabolic substrate for the normal intestinal flora and also for *Diphyllobothrium latum* when this parasite is found to be flourishing abundantly in the small intestine.

Known as the Schilling test, it consists of first giving parenterally a saturation dose of B_{12} so that the radioactive B_{12} given later by mouth will be absorbed in the distal small intestine and eliminated in the urine at the rate of 7 per cent or more of the amount given in 24 hours. Sources of error are vomiting, gastric surgery, stomach disease, and deficiency of intrinsic factor. Vitamin B_{12} must combine with intrinsic factor in the stomach in order to pass into the intestine and be absorbed. In the absence of these errors, a marked decrease in the excretion of B_{12} in the urine indicates malabsorption in the ileum or abnormal growth of bacteria in the small intestine.

Absorption of B_{12} is normal in exocrine pancreatic insufficiency, biliary insufficiency (not secondary to abnormal bacterial proliferation), abetalipoproteinemia, and resection of the jejunum. It is abnormal in all other cases of malabsorption, especially celiac sprue, tropical sprue, abnormal bacterial overgrowth, and diseases or resections of the ileum.

Bile acid breath test

This relatively simple test can be performed in any radioisotope laboratory. By measuring the fate of conjugated bile acids, it supplies valuable information regarding the functional integrity of the terminal ileum or the presence of bacterial overgrowth in the small intestine.

Bile acid conjugated with [^{14}C]glycine or [^{14}C]taurine is administered by mouth. Under normal conditions the conjugated bile salts are absorbed in the ileum, return to the liver, and are re-excreted into the bile. Only a minute fraction of the conjugated bile acid-[^{14}C]glycine reaches the colon, where it is metabolized by the colonic flora to $^{14}CO_2$ and excreted via the lungs. In case of bacterial overgrowth in the small intestine or ileal dysfunction, the bile salts are abnormally deconjugated by bacteria, resulting in a marked increase in excretion of $^{14}CO_2$ in the breath.

Biopsy of the small intestine is the subject of Chapter 23.

Bibliography

Finlay JM, Hogarth J, Wightman KJR: A clinical evaluation of the D-xylose tolerance test. *Ann Intern Med* 61:411, 1964

Fromm H, Hofmann AF: Breath test for altered bile and metabolism. *Lancet* 2:621, 1971

Gray GM: Maldigestion and malabsorption: Clinical manifestations and specific diagnosis. In *Gastrointestinal Disease* (Sleisenger MH, Fordtran JS, eds), 2nd ed, p 272. Philadelphia: Saunders, 1978

Wilson FA, Dietschy JM: Differential diagnostic approach to clinical problems of malabsorption. *Gastroenterology* 61:911, 1971

SUMMARY

The malabsorption syndrome may manifest the typical clinical picture, or with vague digestive complaints or nutritional and metabolic changes. The following studies should be made on all patients: blood carotene, quantitative stool fats, D-xylose absorption, radioactive B_{12} absorption or bile acid breath test, and biopsy of the small intestine.

Biopsy of the small intestine

23

Twenty years ago, peroral biopsy of the small intestine be-
came possible and a great change took place in the understanding and diagnosis of diseases of this important and
previously poorly accessible part of the digestive system. Table 23-1 summarizes the diagnostic value of this procedure.

Even though the biopsy findings are not specific in celiac
sprue, they are especially valuable in the study of this disease, which is the most important disorder causing
malabsorption. In untreated patients, biopsy shows extreme
shortening and even disappearance of the villi as well as simultaneous marked hypertrophy of the crypts. The lamina
propria is heavily infiltrated with lymphocytes, plasma

TABLE 23-1

Diagnostic value of biopsy of the small intestine

Diseases in which biopsy is diagnostic

Whipple's disease	Systemic mastocytosis
Abetalipoproteinemia	Systemic amyloidosis
Immunodeficiency syndromes	Intestinal parasites:
Intestinal lymphoma	giardiasis, coccidiosis,
Intestinal lymphangiectasia	strongyloidiasis,
Eosinophilic enteritis	capillariasis, cryptosporidiosis

Diseases in which biopsy may be abnormal but not diagnostic

Celiac sprue	Radiation enteritis
Tropical sprue	Infectious gastroenteritis
Unclassified sprue	Syndrome of bacterial overgrowth
Folic acid deficiency	Drug-induced enteropathies
Vitamin B_{12} deficiency	Malnutrition

Diseases in which biopsy is normal

Postgastrectomy syndrome	Functional disturbances in the intestine
Exocrine pancreatic insufficiency	Ulcerative colitis
Cirrhosis of the liver	

cells, and often polymorphonuclear leukocytes. When the patient is placed on a gluten-free diet, avoiding wheat, rye, barley, and oats, gradual improvement in the epithelium takes place, until it becomes almost normal.

The dissecting microscope is very useful in studying the normal and pathologic mucosa of the intestine.

Whipple's disease is very rare. It's still important to know the characteristic histologic findings of the disease, since it can be successfully treated with broad-spectrum antibiotics. Biopsy shows very large macrophages infiltrated with periodic acid-Schiff-positive granules of glucoproteins that replace the normal cell elements in the lamina propria and distort the intestinal villi. The lymph vessels of the mucosa and submucosa are dilated and full of fat. Rod-shaped bacilli can be seen in the mucosa in untreated cases by means of the

TABLE 23-2

Laboratory, X-ray, and biopsy findings in

Test	Pancreatic Insufficiency	Biliary Insufficiency	Bacterial overgrowth	Celiac sprue	Tropical sprue	Whipple's disease
Fecal fat	↑ ↑ ↑	↑	↑	↑ ↑	↑ ↑	↑
D-Xylose	N	N	↓	↓	↓	N
Vitamin B_{12}	N	N	↓	↓	↓	N
Biopsy	N	N	N or A	A	±	A
Small bowel X-ray	N	N	N or A	A	±	±

N = normal; A = abnormal.

electron microscope or the high-resolution light microscope. These bacilli have not been fully characterized.

Abetalipoproteinemia and immunodeficiency syndromes are rare and give rise to many varied extraintestinal symptoms as well as to steatorrhea and other manifestations of malabsorption. They are usually diagnosed without intestinal biopsy by finding a lack of beta lipoprotein and gamma globulin, respectively, in the blood. Biopsy shows enormous vacuoles in the cytoplasm of the villous epithelial cells in abetalipoproteinemia. Special stains show the vacuoles to be full of fat. The intestinal cells are incapable of synthesizing beta lipoproteins, which are necessary for the formation of chylomicrons. Thus the absorbed fat cannot be moved toward the lacteal ducts and lymphatic vessels and it accumulates in the intestine. In agammaglobulinemia, there is a marked decrease in number of plasma cells in the mucosa.

Biopsy may help to diagnose only some types of malabsorption because the histologic changes are not uniformly distributed but rather are patchy throughout the intestinal mucosa. Obviously, in these cases, taking multiple biopsies would increase the chances of getting a diagnostic specimen. Conditions with patchy lesions are the following:

Primary diffuse intestinal lymphoma, a rare type, is found principally in Arabs and Sephardic Jews. Biopsy shows infiltration of malignant cells in the lamina propria.

diseases involving intestinal malabsorption

	Intestinal resection				Zollinger-Ellison syndrome	Scleroderma	Gastric surgery
Amyloidosis	Extensive	Jejunal	Ileal	Lymphoma			
↑↓	↑↑↑ ↓	↑ ↓	↑↑ N	↑ ↓	↑ ±	↑ ↓	↑ N
N	↓	N	↓	↓	N or ↓	N or ↓	↓
A	N	N	N	A	N or A	±	N
±	A	A	A	±	N or A	A	N

Intestinal lymphangiectasia is characterized by dilation of lymphatics, replete with macrophages.

Eosinophilic gastroenteritis shows massive infiltration of eosinophils into the lamina propria and submucosa.

Systemic mastocytosis is another rare disease, characterized by mast cell infiltration of the lamina propria.

Systemic amyloidosis, when it involves the small intestine, forms amyloid deposits in the walls of the blood vessels and in the submucosa. Congo red stain and polarized light identify the amyloid deposits.

Regional enteritis may occur in the duodenum. In these rare cases, a lucky biopsy shows noncaseous granulomas, which are characteristic but not pathognomonic of this disease.

Some intestinal parasites, especially *Giardia,* may be diagnosed by biopsy even though stool examinations and duodenal aspirations are negative. Trophozoites are seen adhering to the mucosa and sometimes inside the wall they have invaded.

Hypogammaglobulinemia and dysgammaglobulinemia show on biopsy large hyperplastic lymphoid follicles, decrease in plasma cells in the lamina propria, and, at times, changes in the villi, varying from shortening to advanced atrophy. Giardiasis and hypogammaglobulinemia frequently occur together.

Tropical sprue, folic acid and vitamin B_{12} deficiency, radiation enteritis, infectious enteritis, bacterial overgrowth invading the small intestine, and advanced malnutrition compose a group of intestinal diseases in which biopsy is not justified because the histologic changes are not specific. Tropical sprue shows intestinal lesions similar to those of celiac sprue, but this is not constant. Often, only slight or minimal changes are seen that occur in many "healthy" people living where this disease is endemic.

In postgastrectomy syndromes, pancreatic insufficiency, biliary obstruction, and chronic liver disease, the biopsy is normal. Of course, a normal biopsy is not without importance because it lets you rule out the diseases that have specific lesions.

The tests described here yield not only the diagnosis of malabsorption syndromes but also their exact etiology. Table 23-2 summarizes the characteristics of the most important diseases that involve intestinal malabsorption.

Bibliography

Perera DR, Weinstein WM, Rubin CE: Small intestinal biopsy. *Hum Pathol* 6:157, 1975

Rubin CE, Dobbins WO: Peroral biopsy of the small intestine: A review of its diagnostic usefulness. *Gastroenterology* 49:676, 1965

Shiner M: Duodenal biopsy. *Lancet* 1:17, 1956

Trier JS: Diagnostic value of peroral biopsy of the proximal small intestine. *N Engl J Med* 285:1470, 1971

SUMMARY

There is a host of diseases (see Table 23-1) in which small intestine biopsy is diagnostic, other diseases in which biopsy is abnormal but not pathognomonic, and a variety of conditions in which biopsy is normal. In celiac sprue, the most important derangement causing malabsorption, the biopsy, although not pathognomonic, is significant. The tissue changes gradually return to normal on a gluten-free diet. See Table 23-2 for characteristics of the most important diseases associated with intestinal malabsorption.

Uncommon causes of diarrhea

24

Most of the diseases causing diarrhea have been included in the diagnostic plan suggested. Some diseases that infrequently or only occasionally cause diarrhea need additional studies to establish the diagnosis: hyperthyroidism, adrenal insufficiency, immunodeficiency syndromes, Zollinger-Ellison syndrome, pancreatic cholera, and carcinoid syndrome.

Hyperthyroidism

Diagnosis of hyperthyroidism can be easily made via tests of thyroid function, especially thyroxine (T_4) and triiodothyronine (T_3) concentrations in plasma.

Adrenal insufficiency

If chronic adrenal insufficiency is kept in mind, it can be diagnosed by tests of serum electrolytes, Thorn's test, 24-hour urinary excretion of 17-ketosteroids and 11-hydroxycorticosteroids, and plasma cortisol.

Immunodeficiency syndromes

Primary acquired hypogammaglobulinemia should be suspected if the patient (usually a child or adolescent) has chronic diarrhea, malnutrition, frequent respiratory tract infections, chronic resistant *Giardia* infestation, and/or radiologic evidence of lymphoid nodular hyperplasia of the small bowel. Electrophoretic and immunoelectrophoretic studies of serum proteins will confirm the diagnosis by showing low levels of gamma globulin, IgG, and particularly IgA and IgM.

Zollinger-Ellison syndrome

Zollinger-Ellison syndrome may be easily diagnosed by radioimmunoassay of circulating serum gastrin. Figures usually above 150 pg/ml—frequently above 1,000 pg/ml—are found in this syndrome. (Normal levels are between 20 and 150 pg/ml.) The diagnosis may be suspected if more than 100 mEq of hydrochloric acid are excreted in a nocturnal 12-hour period or if the ratio between basal and maximal histamine-induced secretion is higher than 0.6 : 1. Even a simple test may suggest the diagnosis: The diarrhea will be controlled by continuous gastric aspiration through a nasogastric catheter.

Pancreatic cholera

Pancreatic cholera syndrome is due to pancreatic and other tumors. Victims of this disorder experience chronic, intermittent, profuse, watery diarrhea with dehydration and hypokalemia. Laboratory tests show hypochlorhydria. The diagnosis may be made by measuring the serum concentration of vasoactive intestinal polypeptide (VIP).* Sometimes the pancreatic tumor may be diagnosed by selective arteriography.

Carcinoid syndrome

Diarrhea is one of the chief components. When there is liver metastasis, the diagnosis can be made by measuring the urinary excretion of the serotonin metabolite 5-hydroxyindoleacetic acid. Because its daily excretion is variable, measurements should be done for several days. Another diagnostic procedure is the intravenous injection of 1 μg of epinephrine, which produces the typical facial erythema of the carcinoid syndrome. Finally, the diagnosis can be made at times by X-ray if it shows a filling defect in the ileum associated with an abrupt bend caused by fibrosis of the mesentery (Chapter 20).

Bibliography

Hermans PE, Huizenga KA, Hoffman H, et al: Dysgammaglobulinemia associated with nodular lymphoid hyperplasia of the small intestine. *Am J Med* 40:78, 1966

Hersh T, Floch M, Binder HJ, et al: Disturbance of the jejunal and colonic bacterial flora in immunoglobulin deficiencies. *Am J Clin Nutr* 23:1595, 1970

Jinich H: Diarrea por hipertiroidismo oculto. *Rev Gastroenterol Mex* 24:93, 1959

Said SI, Faloona GD: Elevated plasma and tissue levels of vasoactive intestinal polypeptide in the WDHH syndrome due to pancreatic, bronchogenic and other tumors. *N Engl J Med* 293:155, 1975

Sjoderma A, Melmon KL: The carcinoid spectrum. *Gastroenterology* 47:104, 1964

---

*There are controversies regarding the usefulness of this assay.

SUMMARY

Infrequent causes of diarrhea are hyperthyroidism, which may be readily diagnosed by thyroid function tests (T_4 and T_3); chronic adrenal insufficiency, which shows up on serum electrolyte tests, Thorn's test, 24-hour urinary excretion of 17-ketosteroids and 11-hydroxycorticosteroids, and plasma cortisol; primary acquired hypogammaglobulinemia, which can be detected via electrophoretic and immunoelectrophoretic studies of the serum protein showing low levels of gamma globulins, IgG, IgA, and IgM; Zollinger-Ellison syndrome, which is diagnosed via radioimmunoassay that reveals circulating serum gastrin levels above the normal 150 pg/ml and often above 1,000 pg/ml; pancreatic cholera syndrome, which can be diagnosed by findings of hypochlorhydria, measuring the serum vasoactive intestinal polypeptide (VIP) concentration, and sometimes by selective arteriography that reveals the underlying tumor; and metastatic liver carcinoid, which can be diagnosed from the urinary excretion of 5-hydroxyindoleacetic acid (the serotonin metabolite), facial erythema following IV injection of 1 μg of epinephrine, or typical X-ray findings of a filling defect in the ileum associated with an abrupt bend.

PART III

DIARRHEAL DISEASES

Diarrhea from dietary indiscretion

25

Who of us has not suffered acute diarrhea from unwise eating? Who does not remember in childhood gorging himself on unripe fruit or filling up on too many pastries and sweets, knowing all too well that he would have to pay for his indiscretions with a bellyache and cramps that were alleviated only by frequent, sudden trips to the toilet? The clinical picture is clear: acute diarrhea with frequent liquid stools, gas, and colicky pain. Nausea, vomiting, and abdominal distention often accompany these symptoms. The illness causes no fever, usually lasts a few hours or at the most a couple of days, and subsides without treatment. There is always a history of qualitative or quantitative dietary indiscretion. Treatment consists of a few hours' fast and gradual return to a normal diet, beginning with clear liquids and advancing to low-residue foods such as cereal, tea, lemonade, gelatin, consommé, cooked lean meat, and pureed vegetables.

Probably these diarrheas are of osmotic origin.

Food poisoning

26

Food poisoning is a common cause of acute diarrhea. The onset is sudden, with nausea, vomiting, and abdominal pain. These symptoms are all due to the ingestion of foods containing bacterial, chemical, animal, or vegetable toxins.

Food poisoning without diarrhea but with other symptoms, as occur in botulism, poisoning with fluorides or methyl chloride, poisonous mushrooms, and other toxins that attack the central nervous system, will not be discussed.

Staphylococcus toxin is the most common cause of food poisoning. The clinical history is classical. One to six hours after eating the contaminated food, the patient suddenly begins to feel very sick with nausea and abdominal cramps. Soon he begins to vomit and pass frequent diarrheal stools. The illness is sometimes so severe that hospitalization is necessary. Loss of water and electrolytes makes this a very serious disease in children and old people, who need to be treated promptly with intravenous fluids to restore liquid and electrolyte balance. Usually the disease lasts a few hours, rarely more than six, and stops spontaneously without any treatment except antiemetic and antispasmodic medication and the ingestion, as soon as possible, of abundant liquids.

The disease is not infectious. It's caused by a toxin produced by *Staphylococcus* growing in foods such as cream-filled pastries, custards, cheese, doughnuts, ice cream, milk, meat, sauces, or ham. Common sources of staphylococci are the human nose, skin, and pharynx, from which sites they easily reach the food. Lack of refrigeration then allows the bacteria to grow and produce large quantities of enterotoxin.

Intoxication with *Clostridium perfringens* is more benign and the incubation period longer, eight to 24 hours. The spores are normally found in the stools. Unclean hands contaminate the food which, if kept at 38° to 48°C for several hours, provides a medium for the organisms to grow and produce toxin.

More than 70 varieties of poisonous mushrooms exist. Two of these, *Amanita phalloides* and *Amanita muscaria*, cause acute gastroenteritis as well as choleriform, neurotoxic, and hemolytic syndromes.

A. phalloides produces a toxin that causes sialorrhea, nausea, vomiting, cramps, and profuse diarrhea, which may become hemorrhagic, six to 15 hours after ingestion. Dehydration occurs so suddenly and so severely that it may cause death. Various organs develop parenchymatous lesions, especially the liver, kidneys, and central nervous system. This is caused by the toxin, a thermostable polypeptide. The patient may die in a few days from massive liver cell necrosis.

A. muscaria contains muscarine, a parasympathomimetic alkaloid, as well as variable amounts of a substance that acts on the central nervous system and another parasympatholytic alkaloid. Diarrhea is part of the parasympathetic stimulation, which includes lacrimation, miosis, sweating, sialorrhea, nausea, vomiting, abdominal pain, bronchorrhea, wheezing, bradycardia, and arterial hypotension. Treatment is atropine, 1 to 2 mg every 30 minutes until symptoms subside.

The gastroenterologist should be able to recognize poisoning with arsenic, which is occasionally added to food for criminal or suicidal purposes or by accident, since it occurs in insecticides and rat poison. Acute poisoning causes nausea, vomiting, severe diarrhea, burning of the mouth and throat, and severe abdominal pain. The vomiting is hemorrhagic, and death from circulatory collapse may occur within a few hours. Treatment is immediate gastric lavage, intravenous fluids, blood and plasma, vasopressors, and dimercaprol (British Anti-Lewisite, BAL).

Bibliography

Cohen JO (ed): *The Staphylococci.* New York: Wiley-Interscience, 1972

Committee on Food Protection: *Toxicants Occurring Naturally in Foods,* 2nd ed. Washington, DC: National Academy of Sciences Publication 73.8988, 1973

Goodman LS, Gilman A: *The Pharmacological Basis of Therapeutics,* 5th ed. New York: Macmillan, 1975

Grady GF, Keusch GT: Pathogenesis of bacterial diarrhea. *N Engl J Med* 285:831, 1971

SUMMARY

Food containing bacterial, chemical, animal, or vegetable toxins may cause nausea, vomiting, abdominal pain, and acute diarrhea. Among the most common is *Staphylococcus* toxin. The symptoms come on one to six hours after eating the food. They are severe; loss of water and electrolytes may represent an emergency. Liquid replacement, antiemetics, and antispasmodics are the treatment. *Clostridium perfringens* intoxication is less severe, comes on eight to 24 hours after eating, and is due to unclean hands' contaminating the food.

More than 70 varieties of poisonous mushrooms exist. *Amanita phalloides* and *Amanita muscaria* cause acute gastroenteritis and neurologic and hematologic symptoms. *A. phalloides* toxin causes salivation, nausea, vomiting, cramps, marked diarrhea at times with blood, severe dehydration, and sometimes death. The liver may be seriously necrosed, causing death in a few days. *A. muscaria* toxin is muscarine, a parasympathetic alkaloid. Treatment is 1 to 2 mg of atropine every 30 minutes until symptoms subside.

Arsenic is still used homicidally or suicidally. The symptoms are nausea, vomiting, severe diarrhea, burning mouth and throat, and severe abdominal pain. Treatment is immediate gastric lavage, IV fluids, blood and plasma, vasopressors, and BAL.

Acute bacterial diarrhea

Epidemiology

27

Many criteria enter into the classification of a country as underdeveloped. One of the most important of these, some believe, is the high incidence of morbidity and mortality from acute infectious gastroenteritis. This is an unfailing indication of poor hygiene and sanitation with consequent fecal contamination of food and water. Unfortunately, Mexico and the majority of Latin American countries fall into this category. The mortality from enteritis in the United States in 1968 was 1.5 per 100,000 inhabitants, compared with 145 per 100,000 in the Federal District in Mexico. At the Children's Hospital in Mexico City, gastroenteritis heads the list of illnesses, with an average of 9,000 cases per year, or approximately 20 per cent of admissions. It has been stated that diarrheas of bacterial etiology are the single greatest cause of mortality in underdeveloped areas of the world and that in any given 24-hour period 200 million people on earth are suffering from gastroenteritis.

Shigella, Salmonella, and *Escherichia coli* are the principal bacteria involved. The previously held idea that *Vibrio cholerae* was nonexistent in North America has proven incorrect. A case of cholera was discovered in Louisiana in 1978, and an investigation led to detection of 10 other *V. cholerae* 01 infections. It was determined that the vehicle of transmission was cooked crabs from the Louisiana marshes, and evidence was found suggesting that similar organisms had persisted undetected along the Gulf Coast for at least five years. Other organisms of limited importance also causing bacterial diarrhea are *Staphylococcus aureus, Clostridium, Vibrio, Yersinia, Pseudomonas, Proteus,* and *Klebsiella.*

Bacterial infections can be divided into three groups on the basis of their pathogenesis:

1. Bacteria that do not invade tissues but multiply in the lumen of the gut, producing exotoxins that cause the diarrhea (Chapter 2): *V. cholerae, Shigella dysenteriae,* and some toxigenic strains of *E. coli*
2. Bacteria that invade the intestinal mucosa, causing inflammation and ulcers: shigellae and some "invasive" *E. coli*
3. Invasive agents that penetrate into the cells of the intestinal mucosa but do not cause any ulceration or necrosis: salmonellae belong to this group.

Some *Salmonella* species, such as those responsible for typhoid fever, cause an inflammatory reaction with mononuclear cells in the lamina propria and invade the bloodstream. Other salmonellae are known to give rise to an inflammatory reaction with polymorphonuclear cells and in those cases the infection remains confined to the intestinal mucosa; these patients develop acute gastroenteritis, with diarrhea being the chief symptom.

Shigella species

Shigella organisms are considered to be the most frequent cause of infectious diarrhea. *S. flexneri* predominates in areas with deficient sanitation, while in other areas *S. sonnei, boydii,* and *dysenteriae* species are more prevalent.

Shigellae are immobile bacteria that ferment glucose without gas production but do not ferment lactose in a 24-hour period. They have other biochemical reactions characteristic of the genus. They produce two kinds of somatic antigens or endotoxins, one specific for the genus and the other specific for the type or species. All species of *Shigella* are pathogenic for humans because of their invasive properties. The bacteria penetrate the epithelial cells by pinocytosis, reach the lamina propria, there produce an inflammatory reaction with polymorphonuclear infiltration, and finally, because of the accumulation of metabolites and the liberation of endotoxins, give rise to hypoxia and other conditions favoring the formation of ulcers. The most severe lesions are in the rectum and descending colon, decreasing proximally along the length of the colon. Besides the invasive properties of these organisms, at least one species, *S. dysenteriae* (and perhaps others), produces enterotoxins that are capable of inducing small-intestinal secretion of isotonic fluid in a manner similar to cholera enterotoxin. *Shigella* infection is extremely rare in newborns. Its incidence increases progressively to a maximum at two years.

Shigella infection is spread by fecal contamination from patients ill with the disease or from carriers, directly from person to person or through contamination of foods and drinks by food handlers or insects that come in contact with feces and then carry the bacteria to foods. Once the patient becomes infected, he begins to expel the bacteria in his feces. These organisms disappear during convalescence except in unusual cases, where they continue to be present for longer periods, leading to a carrier state.

The widespread belief, even among physicians, that water is important in the spread of diarrheal infections has given rise to the expression "water-borne diseases." Water is not a favorable medium for either the survival or the multiplica-

tion of bacteria, since it tends to dilute them. The only exceptions to this are in the transmission of *Salmonella typhi* and
V. cholerae.

Salmonella species

Salmonellae are motile bacteria with characteristic reactions, among which are the fermentation of glucose with
formation of gas. They are unable to ferment lactose or hydrolyze urea. Their antigenic structure is complex and includes two principal antigens, the somatic antigens or endotoxins, called O, and the flagellar antigen, called H. Some
serotypes also have a capsular antigen, called K or Vi. The
Salmonella genus is divided into 10 groups and more than
1,400 serotypes, all pathogenic for humans, animals, or
both. They have great invasive power, so that, like shigellae,
they penetrate epithelial cells but, unlike shigellae, do not
destroy these cells or cause ulceration. They do, however,
cause an inflammatory reaction in the lamina propria,
whose severity depends on whether the infection is localized
or generalized. If the inflammatory reaction is mononuclear, the circulation is invaded and a typhoid or bacteremic
syndrome is produced. If the inflammatory reaction is
polymorphonuclear, the infection is confined to the mucosa
and causes acute gastroenteritis.

The relationship between underdeveloped countries and
gastroenteritis does not apply to *Salmonella* infections. In
fact, *Salmonella* infections have markedly increased in
highly developed countries in the last 10 to 15 years, apparently because of massive industrialization and distribution
of food products. In contrast to *Shigella* and other
enteropathogens that infect humans only, many serotypes
of *Salmonella* also infect animals, including domestic fowl,
swine, cattle, horses, dogs, cats, rats, mice, toads, frogs,
and turtles.

Human beings, whether or not made ill by *Salmonella*, can
be carriers for weeks, months, and even years and can excrete the bacteria in their feces indefinitely. It's evident,
then, that infection may be spread by direct contact from
person to person or by ingesting insufficiently cooked meat,

viscera, or eggs of infected animals. Refrigeration retards growth but does not destroy *Salmonella*. Water can be made potable by adding chlorine, 1 mg/liter.

Escherichia coli

The different serologic types of *E. coli* are motile, ferment glucose and lactose with formation of gas, and give biochemical reactions characteristic of the genus. They have three kinds of antigens: somatic or endotoxins, or O; flagellar, or H; and capsular, or K. More than 148 O antigens, 51 H antigens, and 92 K antigens have been described, corresponding to several hundred serotypes. Recent evidence challenges the serologic basis of identifying pathogenic strains of *E. coli* and suggests that routine serogrouping of these bacteria in sporadic cases of diarrhea, using commercial antisera currently available, is useless for practical purposes. The diagnosis of "enteropathogenic *E. coli* diarrhea" is unreliable when the evidence is based solely on serologic identification.

Recently, two groups of *E. coli* pathogenic to both children and adults have been described. One group produces an enterotoxin similar in action to *V. cholerae.* The other group, like *Shigella,* invades the intestinal mucosa. It is very likely that these groups of *E. coli,* especially those producing enterotoxin, could be responsible for many cases of tourist diarrhea (Chapter 33).

The various strains of *E. coli* are often found in the intestines of healthy children and adults, and these individuals may therefore be carriers. The number of bacteria expelled in their feces, however, is generally small, so they're not important in the transmission of the disease. However, year-old infants infected with pathogenic *E. coli* eliminate great quantities of the organism, especially during the first 48 hours of infection, readily passing it to other children either by direct contact or by contaminated fomites and even by means of small amounts of airborne fecal matter. It's easy to understand the danger of hospital epidemics in wards containing newborns and older infants, and the necessity for strict sanitary controls as soon as such a case is discovered.

The bacteria can remain viable in dust for as long as 27 days. The infection can be transmitted from the mother to the new-born infant through the placenta in cases of bacteremia, and by fecal contamination at birth. Invasive *E. coli* has been shown to be an important cause of endemic diarrhea in the United States.

Campylobacter fetus

Campylobacter fetus has been recently recognized to cause diarrheal disease in humans, producing a typical clinical syndrome with acute onset of diarrhea, abdominal pain, fever, and constitutional symptoms. Stool examination reveals blood and polymorphonuclear leukocytes in a high percentage of patients. The diagnosis may be established by stool culture or by a 4-fold rise in antibody titers to the organism. The organism is sensitive to erythromycin, but the illness is largely self-limited. Poultry, dogs, unpasteurized milk, food, and infected children may spread this infection.

Symptomatology

The clinical pictures of acute infectious diarrhea caused by *Shigella, Salmonella, E. coli,* and *Campylobacter* are similar enough to be described jointly, pointing out what differences exist. In clinical practice it is very difficult to make an etiologic diagnosis of diarrhea without laboratory tests. The principal symptom is diarrhea of sudden onset, sometimes preceded by nausea, vomiting, malaise, diffuse, colicky abdominal pain, and fever. The fever is transitory and usually subsides within 24 to 48 hours. Stools are liquid, numbering five to 20 or more a day, and the desire to defecate is urgent. In *Shigella* and sometimes *Salmonella* infections, the stools may contain mucus and blood. Tenesmus is not unusual.

In mild forms there may be only anorexia, low-grade fever, and three or four semiliquid bowel movements a day. More severe cases, however, cause high fever, frequent vomiting, especially in infants, and very frequent stools, resulting in dehydration, hydroelectrolytic imbalance, shock, and acute renal failure in very severe cases. These complications are rare in older children and adults, but they are a danger in infants, young children, and old people.

Treatment

Treatment consists of rehydration of the patient to restore the fluid and electrolyte balance. Antiemetic medication is justified if vomiting interferes with oral ingestion and retention of fluids. Only low-residue foods should be given. The abuse of antidiarrheal medication is unwise. Clinical experience has shown that recovery is more rapid and complete if the diarrhea is not stopped prematurely. Interfering with the motility of the intestine favors bacterial proliferation and invasion. Rapid emptying of the bowel in diarrhea is a defense mechanism: The body protects itself against the intestinal invasion by decreasing contact time between the bacteria and mucosal cells.

Antibiotics have not been shown to be of value in *Salmonella* gastroenteritis; quite the contrary. Treatment with chloramphenicol or ampicillin prolongs the period of excretion of *Salmonella* during convalescence and favors the development of organisms resistant to these antibiotics. Infections with these organisms are usually mild and self-limiting. Prompt and complete recovery takes place if hydroelectrolytic equilibrium is maintained.

In infections with *Shigella* and enteropathogenic *E. coli,* intense and indiscriminate use of antibiotics has resulted in the development of many resistant strains. This resistance is due to transferable R factors. R factors can be transferred to shigellae or other pathogenic bacteria through nonpathogenic *E. coli* or other gram-negative bacteria. Thus, if a person ingests one of these R-positive bacteria and the R factor is transferred to his intestinal flora, and if he later becomes infected with *Shigella* or enteropathogenic *E. coli* that are susceptible to various antibiotics, the R factor can make these bacteria resistant.

In the majority of cases in children as well as in adults, infections with *Shigella,* like those with *Salmonella,* tend to be self-limiting. There is the additional advantage that the invasiveness and pathogenicity of *Shigella* on entering the circulation is less than with *Salmonella*. For that reason, it is desirable to repress the impulse to administer antibiotics unless the clinical picture is severe enough to justify their use. Sensitivity tests in vitro are needed to choose the right antibiotic. Sulfonamides and tetracyclines are no longer effective, and many strains have developed resistance to ampicillin, chloramphenicol, and sulfamethoxazole-trimethoprim, which used to be very effective.

Benign infections with pathogenic *E. coli* require no antibiotic therapy. This should be reserved for serious cases with septicemia, shock, and other complications.

Bibliography

Aserloff B, Bennett JV: Effect of antibiotic therapy in acute salmonellosis on the fecal excretion of salmonellae. *N Engl J Med* 281:636, 1969

Blake PA, Allegra DT, Snyder JD, et al: Cholera—A possible endemic focus in the United States. *N Engl J Med* 302:365, 1980

Blasser MJ, Berkowitz ID, LaForce FM, et al: Campylobacter enteritis: Clinical and epidemiological features. *Ann Intern Med* 91:179, 1979

Charney AN, Gots RE, Formal SB, et al: Activation of intestinal mucosal adenylate cyclase by Shigella dysenteriae I enterotoxin. *Gastroenterology* 70:1085, 1976

DuPont HL: Editorial. Etiologic diagnosis of acute diarrhea. *Ann Intern Med* 88:707, 1978

DuPont HL, Hornick RB: Adverse effect of Lomotil therapy in shigellosis. *JAMA* 226:1525, 1973

DuPont HL, Formal SB, Hornick RB, et al: Pathogenesis of E. coli diarrhea. *N Engl J Med* 285:1, 1971

Field M: New strategies for treating watery diarrhea. *N Engl J Med* 297:1121, 1977

Fineberg L: The management of the critically ill child with dehydration secondary to diarrhea. *Pediatrics* 45:1029, 1970

Gangarosa EJ, Merson MH: Epidemiologic assessment of the relevance of the so-called enteropathogenic serogroups of E. coli in diarrhea. *N Engl J Med* 296:1210, 1977

Gorbach SL: Acute diarrhea—A "toxin" disease. *N Engl J Med* 283:44, 1970

Grady GF, Keusch GT: Pathogenesis of bacterial diarrheas. *N Engl J Med* 285:831, 1971

Harris JC, DuPont HL, Hornick RB: Fecal leukocytes in diarrheal illness. *Ann Intern Med* 76:697, 1972

Pickering LK, DuPont HL, Olarte J: Single-dose tetracycline therapy for shigellosis in adults. *JAMA* 239:853, 1978

Ryder RW, Wacksmuth IK, Buxton AE, et al: Infantile diarrhea produced by heat-stable enterotoxigenic Escherichia coli. *N Engl J Med* 295:849, 1976

Weissman JB, Gangarosa EJ, DuPont HL, et al: Shigellosis. To treat or not to treat. *JAMA* 229:1215, 1974

SUMMARY

Bacterial diarrhea is said to be the largest single cause of death in underdeveloped countries. In any given 24-hour period 200 million people on earth have gastroenteritis due mostly to *Shigella, Salmonella,* and *Escherichia coli.* Pathologically, bacterial infections can be divided into three major groups: where the bacteria multiply in the lumen, producing endotoxins, but do not invade tissues, typical of the cholera vibrio, *Shigella dysenteriae,* and toxigenic strains of *E. coli;* where bacteria invade the intestinal mucosa, causing inflammation and ulcers, typical of shigellae and some invasive *E. coli;* and where bacteria invade intestinal mucosal cells but do not cause ulceration or necrosis, typical of *Salmonella,* some entering the bloodstream and others confined to the mucosa.

Shigellae are the most frequent cause of infectious diarrhea. They are all pathogenic for humans, producing two types of endotoxin, and are invasive, often causing intestinal ulceration, particularly in the rectum and descending colon. Shigellosis is rare in newborns, but incidence increases up to two years. Infection is spread by fecal contamination. Water is not a vector of diarrheal infection except that produced by *Salmonella typhi.*

Salmonella comprises 10 groups and more than 1,400 serotypes, all pathogenic for humans and animals. They are highly invasive but cause no ulceration. They may enter the circulation and produce a typhoid or bacteremic syndrome. When confined to the mucosa, they produce acute gastroenteritis. Salmonellosis has increased markedly in highly developed countries in recent years. Humans can be carriers for years. Water can be made potable by adding 1 mg of chlorine per liter.

E. coli have several hundred serotypes. Two groups are pathogenic for both adults and children. One produces an enterotoxin and acts like the cholera vibrio; the other invades the intestinal mucosa like *Shigella*. These may be responsible for tourist diarrhea. Humans may be carriers at any age, but it is the year-old infant carrier who is responsible for spread.

Campylobacter fetus may cause acute diarrhea in humans. Stools show blood and white cells. Stool culture and a 4-fold rise in antibody titers are diagnostic. Erythromycin is effective, but most often not necessary.

Acute infectious diarrheas due to *Shigella, Salmonella,* or *E. coli* present similar pictures with some minor differences. Etiologic diagnosis must be made by laboratory tests. Severe diarrhea and vomiting may result in dehydration, electrolyte imbalance, shock, and renal failure, especially in infants. Treatment consists of rehydration, with antiemetics if vomiting is severe. Overmedication must be avoided. Recovery is more rapid if the diarrhea is not stopped prematurely. Antibiotics are of no value in *Salmonella* infections, which are usually mild and self-limiting. *Shigella* and *E. coli* enteropathogens have produced many resistant strains. If the condition is serious, antibiotic sensitivity tests are in order to choose the proper antibiotic.

Cholera and other vibrio infections

28

Seven cholera pandemics have occurred in the last two centuries. The seventh pandemic began 20 years ago in Indonesia, spread through South and Southeast Asia, the Middle East, Africa, and parts of Europe, and continues to the present time. As mentioned in Chapter 27, an endemic focus was recently discovered in the Louisiana marshes. The increase in air travel to all parts of the world makes it necessary for physicians to be alert and to know how to diagnose and treat this fearful disease.

Cholera is caused by *Vibrio cholerae*, a gram-negative bacillus, aerobic, curved, and motile by means of its flagella. Contaminated water and food spread the disease. The organism can live in the gallbladders of healthy carriers. These persons are the reservoirs of the bacillus and are probably responsible for epidemics and for its continued survival in endemic areas such as the delta of the river Ganges.

Vibrio cholerae

V. cholerae produces an exotoxin that rapidly binds to small-bowel mucosa and stimulates adenylate cyclase in the epithelial cells. The resulting increase in intracellular cyclic adenosine 3',5'-monophosphate leads to the secretion of enormous amounts of isotonic solutions in all parts of the small intestine without producing any histologic changes in the epithelium or in the endothelium of the blood capillaries. The stools contain sodium and chloride in the same concentrations as plasma, while the concentration of bicarbonate is double and that of potassium is three to five times higher than in plasma. The patient may pass as much as 1 liter of liquid stool per hour. It's easy, then, to understand how this profuse diarrhea puts the patient in great danger of severe dehydration, electrolyte imbalance, shock, metabolic acidosis, hyponatremia, renal insufficiency, uremia, and death.

The diagnosis is not difficult where the disease is endemic or during an epidemic. *V. cholerae* can be identified in cultures or by microscopic examination either with immunofluorescence, phase contrast microscopy, or dark-field illumination after immobilizing the vibrio with specific antiserum. A high index of suspicion is mandatory in any patient with severe secretory diarrhea. Rectal swabs should be obtained and bacteriology laboratories should be encouraged to use thiosulfate-citrate-bile salts-sucrose (TCBS) agar in culturing diarrheal stools.

Prompt diagnosis and treatment reduce the mortality almost to zero. The organism is sensitive to tetracycline, chloramphenicol, and furazolidone (Furoxone). These drugs will shorten the course of the disease and reduce the volume of stools. But the most important and urgent part of the treatment is rapid fluid replacement by means of IV isotonic saline and bicarbonate, given as fast as 100 ml/minute, in order to maintain a good pulse, skin turgor, and satisfactory diuresis. Control by measuring venous pressure helps prevent overloading the circulation and causing acute pulmonary edema or, on the other hand, being timid and giving too little fluid too slowly. A dramatic therapeutic success was attained a decade ago when it was demonstrated that intestinal absorption of sodium and water is possible in spite of the severe secretory diarrhea of cholera and that absorption is favored by the simultaneous oral administration of glucose.

Other pathogenic vibrios

Besides *V. cholerae,* three other distinct groups of vibrios are now known to be associated with human disease: "noncholera vibrios," *Campylobacter fetus,* and halophilic vibrios, including *V. parahemolyticus* and *V. alginolyticus.*

V. parahemolyticus is now known to be the leading cause of acute diarrheal illness in Japan and has recently been incriminated in many outbreaks of diarrhea in coastal areas of the United States. The illness usually begins acutely with explosive watery diarrhea and abdominal pain but subsides in 24 to 48 hours. The outbreaks have been related to ingestion of inadequately cooked seafood, usually shrimp.

V. alginolyticus has not been incriminated in outbreaks of gastroenteritis.

Bibliography

Blake PA, Allegra DT, Snyder JD, et al: Cholera—A possible endemic focus in the United States. *N Engl J Med* 302:305, 1980

Bolen JL, Zamiska SH, Greenough WB: Clinical features of enteritis due to Vibrio parahemolyticus. *Am J Med* 57:638, 1974

Skirrow MB: Campylobacter enteritis: A "new" disease. *Br Med J* 2:9, 1977

SUMMARY

Cholera, caused by *Vibrio cholerae,* is spread by contaminated water and food and because of greatly increased worldwide travel is now found universally, even in the

United States. *V. cholerae* exotoxin causes excessive liquid
stools, often up to 1 liter/hour, endangering the patient with
shock and death. The organism can be identified on culture
or microscopic examination. Prompt treatment almost always cures and consists primarily of rapid rehydration and
IV bicarbonate. Occasionally tetracycline, chloramphenicol,
and/or furazolidone (Furoxone) may be necessary. Three
other noncholera vibrios are known to affect humans:
Campylobacter fetus and two halophilic vibrios, *V. parahemolyticus* and *V. alginolyticus. V. parahemolyticus* is the
leading cause of diarrhea in Japan and has been involved in
outbreaks in coastal areas in the United States. It is due to
ingestion of inadequately cooked seafood, usually shrimp.

Acute viral gastroenteritis

29

Diarrhea is associated with a number of viral infections, such as poliomyelitis, measles, infectious hepatitis, mumps, and influenza. In these diseases diarrhea is, of course, a symptom of secondary importance. Enteroviruses, on the other hand, cause surprisingly few gastrointestinal symptoms and have rarely been incriminated as major causes of diarrheal disease except for occasional epidemics in infants. In 1973 a new virus, now commonly called a rotavirus, was identified in children with diarrhea. These agents are associated with approximately half of the worldwide, wintertime, nonbacterial gastroenteritis cases in children younger than 3 years. Adults are also susceptible. Smaller, parvovirus-like agents, such as the Norwalk agent, produce periodic, brief community outbreaks with high attack rates affecting children and adults.

Rotaviruses may be identified in fecal suspensions with the help of electron microscopy. Other useful diagnostic procedures are serologic: contraimmune electrophoresis, complement fixation, and enzyme-linked immunosorbent assay (ELISA). These viruses are probably responsible for 30 to 50 per cent of pediatric diarrheas. Parvoviruses are smaller (27 nm as against 70 nm for the rotaviruses) and may be identified in the feces with the help of immune electron microscopy. They induce morphologic and functional changes in the jejunum. The epithelial cells are penetrated by the viral pathogens with resulting inflammation, villus shortening, crypt hypertrophy, increased mitosis, dilation of endoplasmic reticulum, and an increase in intracellular multivesiculate bodies. Brush border enzyme activities are decreased.

Acute viral gastroenteritis lasts about 48 hours with diarrhea, nausea, vomiting, moderately severe colicky abdominal pain, headache, and malaise. It appears especially in epidemics but may persist endemically and be responsible for localized outbreaks and even sporadic cases.

Treatment should be symptomatic. The prognosis is favorable, since the disease subsides spontaneously in less than 72 hours. As with patients who have had an acute bacterial diarrhea, the viral infection may be followed by a temporary malabsorption syndrome with diarrhea, steatorrhea, and meteorism, which can be diagnosed by abnormal D-xylose and lactose absorption tests and increased fat in the stools.

Bibliography

Agus SG, Dolin R, Wyath RG, et al: Acute infectious nonbacterial gastroenteritis. *Ann Intern Med* 79:18, 1973

Bishop RF, Davidson GP, Holmes IH, et al: Viral particles in epithelial cells of duodenal mucosa from children with acute non-bacterial gastroenteritis. *Lancet* 2:1281, 1973

Blacklow NR, Cukor G: Viral gastroenteritis. *N Engl J Med* 304:397, 1981

Davidson GP, Bishop RF, Townley RR, et al: Importance of a new virus in acute sporadic enteritis in children. *Lancet* 1:242, 1975

Kapikian AZ, Kim HW, Wyatt RG, et al: Human reovirus-like agent as the major pathogen associated with "winter" gastroenteritis in hospitalized infants and young adults. *N Engl J Med* 294:965, 1976

Pickering LK, Evans DJ, Munoz O, et al: Prospective study of enteropathogens in children with diarrhea in Houston and Mexico. *J Pediatr* 93:383, 1978

SUMMARY

Diarrhea may be associated with systemic viral diseases. A rotavirus is responsible for one-half the wintertime, nonbacterial gastroenteritis in children under 3. Adults may be involved also. The Norwalk agent, a small parvovirus, causes brief outbreaks of diarrhea. These gastroenteritides are generally short-lived. Treatment is symptomatic.

Intestinal amebiasis

30

Without a doubt, intestinal amebiasis is the most important intestinal disease caused by parasites, and it is certainly one of the most important causes of intestinal symptoms, especially diarrhea.

Since amebae can live in the human intestine without causing any structural changes or symptoms, the term "invasive amebiasis" is preferable for those conditions where the parasite is truly pathogenic. It is important to emphasize that *Entamoeba histolytica* is not an obligatory parasite of man but may often live commensally in the form called "precystic" or "tetragenous." On occasion, however, the ameba may change and grow in size, becoming invasive and losing its ability to form cysts. The reason for this change is not known.

E. histolytica is found throughout the world and is endemic in the wide band of territory between parallels 40 north and 30 south. Probably at least 20 per cent of the world population harbors this parasite. In Ecuador the incidence is 65 per cent, in the United States 5 per cent, and in Mexico 20 per cent. These figures do not, however, represent morbidity, which may be quite different.

Pathogenesis of invasive amebiasis

Some countries, Mexico among them, have a higher incidence of invasive amebiasis than others. In invasive amebiasis the trophozoites penetrate the epithelium of the large intestine and reach the submucosa by means of their motility and their proteolytic enzymes. There they create small areas of gelatinous necrosis (abscesses), which form ulcers when they open into the intestinal lumen. From here the sequence of events depends on the parasite's aggressiveness and the host's regenerative powers. Usually the ulcers remain small and even microscopic, but in some cases the amebae penetrate further and form large ulcers. This is followed by secondary bacterial invasion. The mucosa between the ulcers does not become inflamed but remains normal. The muscular wall is relatively resistant but in severe cases it, as well as the serosa, may be penetrated with consequent perforation and peritonitis. The absence of polymorphonuclear infiltration in both intestinal and hepatic lesions is characteristic.

The intestinal lesions are found all along the colon but are rare in the terminal ileum. The walls thicken especially in the submucosa. The mucosa appears to be affected by a hemorrhagic catarrh. Hemispheric areas of infiltration are surrounded by hyperemia or hemorrhage. Destructive lesions vary from superficial erosions to crater-like ulcers with excavated borders and large ulcers with irregular borders whose base is formed by the muscle layer or even by peritoneum. These big ulcers result from coalescence of several small adjoining ulcers and form submucosal communications with later sloughing of the mucosa. The most typical amebic ulcers have the form of "collar buttons" because of undermining of the submucosa.

Since amebae may live commensally in the human intestine, the finding of their cysts in the stools is no proof of disease. Very frequently patients with irritable colon or another disease of the digestive tract receive vigorous, prolonged antiamebic treatment because cysts were found in their stools. The treatment is based on erroneously ascribing the symptoms to amebiasis when other diseases are responsible. The pathogenicity of *E. histolytica* is considerable, but without question it is the most maligned organism in history.

Clinical forms of amebiasis

The five clinical forms of intestinal amebiasis are acute ulcerative proctocolitis, fulminating colitis, typhloappendicitis, ameboma, and chronic colitis.

Acute amebic ulcerative proctocolitis

This is manifested clinically by the dysenteric syndrome, with its three characteristic symptoms: mucosanguineous stools, colicky low abdominal pain, and tenesmus. The onset is usually sudden, sometimes following a meal rich in irritating foods and alcohol, and lasting only a short time. It may get better and even disappear spontaneously in a few days. In other cases it may become chronic and refractory to the most vigorous treatment. Relapses may occur, or the attack may be followed only by dyspepsia of variable duration.

Characteristic changes are seen by proctosigmoidoscopy (Chapter 15). The typical lesions can be seen even during spontaneous clinical remissions. It isn't unusual to see these lesions in patients who haven't even had the dysentery syndrome but who complain of other symptoms, such as rectal bleeding.

The diagnosis of acute amebic ulcerative proctocolitis is based on the proctosigmoidoscopic findings plus the identification of *E. histolytica* trophozoites in material obtained during the examination or in fresh stools studied immedi-

ately on a warm stage (Chapter 16). Generally, the endoscopic picture is so characteristic that there are few possibilities of diagnostic error. Nevertheless, other diseases
must be taken into account. Granulomatous colitis or
Crohn's disease of the colon, when it involves the rectum, is
seen as small, discrete, punched-out ulcers separated by
normal mucosa, or as deep ulcers that look like those in
amebiasis, often fusiform and following the long axis of the
intestine. Ischemic proctocolitis may also develop rectal
ulcers. Much emphasis has been placed on the perfectly normal mucosa between the ulcers in amebiasis, but this is not
always true. Sometimes all the mucosa is hyperemic and friable and the differential diagnosis from nonspecific ulcerative colitis becomes very difficult—even more so when
antiamebic treatment is unsuccessful. When treatment is
unsuccessful the endoscopic picture does not improve and
the trophozoites of *E. histolytica* may persist in the lesions.

In acute colitis caused by *Shigella,* the mucosa is red,
edematous, friable, and dotted with superficial ulcers. In
dysentery caused by *Schistosoma mansoni,* the mucosa is
thickened and ulcerated with papillomatous excrescences.

The confusion of the differential diagnosis by so many
similar endoscopic pictures should emphasize the necessity
of finding amebic trophozoites in fresh stools. Unless *E.
histolytica* trophozoites are found, the diagnosis is in doubt.
Fortunately, the indirect hemagglutination reaction is positive in at least 80 per cent of cases of invasive amebiasis of
the intestine or liver (Chapter 17).

Fulminating colitis

Fulminating colitis is a very serious disease with numerous
mucosanguineous stools, constant tenesmus, intense constant abdominal pain, high fever, tachycardia, and low
blood pressure. The patient looks dehydrated and toxic. The
abdomen is markedly tender to palpation and may even
show frank signs of generalized acute peritonitis. Laboratory studies show marked leukocytosis, hyponatremia, and
hypokalemia. A flat film of the abdomen shows megacolon,
paralytic ileus, and, in cases of perforation, free intraperi-
toneal air. Proctoscopy reveals extensive amebic ulcers.

Proctoscopy must be done with extreme care in these very sick patients.

Amebic typhloappendicitis

Amebic typhloappendicitis is so-called because of its location in the cecum and the cecal appendix. It is not common. It may be confused with ordinary appendicitis; a differential diagnosis is practically impossible. If the onset is gradual, the accompanying diarrhea and presence of amebae in the stools can warn you of typhloappendicitis so that you can try a therapeutic test, which should solve the problem. This unfortunately is possible only in subacute, relatively mild cases, which are in the minority.

Ameboma

Ameboma of the colon is an inflammatory swelling of the mucosa and submucosa that occurs in amebic colitis and may be confused with malignant tumors or proliferative tuberculosis of the colon. Differential diagnosis is often possible only after surgery followed by microscopic examination of the tissues.

Chronic amebic colitis

Chronic amebic colitis is one of the most common diagnoses made in patients who suffer from chronic colonic symptoms, such as diarrhea, constipation, pain, and flatulence, and who have or have had in the past cysts of *E. histolytica* in the stools. In a large proportion of such cases, this diagnosis is unfounded and the patient suffers from either an irritable colon syndrome, lactose intolerance, or some other disease that causes the same symptoms. Nevertheless, many general practitioners persist in the diagnosis of amebic colitis and blame the failure of treatment on the resistance of the amebae to the medication and to recurrent reinfestation. Such physicians likewise may blame a series of negative laboratory reports on the technical difficulty of finding amebae in the stools.

If so many such cases are not really amebic colitis, the next question is: Does such an entity exist? Many eminent clinicians deny it and state that amebiasis of the colon can be diagnosed only on the basis of invasion by *E. histolytica;* consequently, they say, individuals who pass cysts in their stools and who have no clinical, radiologic, or endoscopic signs of disease, and in whom serologic reactions, correctly interpreted, do not indicate tissue invasion, should be considered to be carriers of *E. histolytica.* This is a controversial subject and the last word probably has not been said. But the practical conclusion is important: On finding cysts of *E. histolytica* in the stools, you should not be content with the diagnosis of chronic amebic colitis but should try to find organic lesions caused by amebae. If you do not find them, you should look for other possible causes of the symptoms. This does not mean you should withhold antiamebic treatment if you find amebae in either the vegetative or the cystic form. But keep in mind that (1) the controversy over chronic amebic colitis has not been settled yet, (2) noninvasive amebae may change at any time to the invasive type in carriers, and (3) carriers of amebae should obviously receive treatment for epidemiologic reasons.

Treatment

Treatment of the asymptomatic patient passing cysts has usually consisted of iodoquinol (diiodohydroxyquin, Panaquin), 650 mg orally three times a day for 20 days. However, it has been effective in only 70 per cent of cases. Furthermore, there has been persistent concern that, like its analogue iodochlorhydroxyquin, it may cause subacute myeloptic neuropathy. Therefore it has been suggested that diloxanide furoate (Furamide) should now be the drug of choice. It is well tolerated and has minimal toxicity.

The drug of choice for invasive (intestinal and extraintestinal) amebiasis is metronidazole (Flagyl), 750 mg three times a day for five to 10 days. In spite of concern about carcinogenicity in rats, its mutagenic action on bacteria, and its extensive use in women with trichomoniasis, there is no evidence of any oncogenic effect in human beings. It produces a metallic taste and occasional nausea, flatulence, and diarrhea. Furthermore, alcoholic drinks should be forbidden during the period of therapy because of the drug's disulfiram-like (Antabuse) effect.

Another drug of comparable efficacy, but more toxic, is emetine, which should be administered by deep intramuscular injection at the dose of 1 mg/kg of body weight daily for five to 10 days, depending on the severity of the clinical picture. Dehydroemetine appears to be as effective as emetine and may have less cardiac toxicity. However, neither drug should be used in patients with known cardiac disease.

Bibliography

Brooke MM: Epidemiology of amebiasis in the U.S. *JAMA* 188:519, 1964

Kean BH: The treatment of amebiasis, a recurrent agony. *JAMA* 235:501, 1976

Krogstad DJ, Spencer HC, Healy GR: Current concepts in parasitology. Amebiasis. *N Engl J Med* 298:262, 1978

Milgran EA, Healy GR, Kagan IG: Studies on the use of the indirect hemagglutination reaction in the diagnosis of amebiasis. *Gastroenterology* 50:645, 1966

Sepulveda B: La amibiasis invasora por Entamoeba histolytica. *Gac Med Mex* 100:201, 1970

Sodeman WA Jr: Amebiasis (clinical seminar). *Am J Dig Dis* 16:51, 1971

Turner JA, Lewis WP, Hayes M, et al: Amebiasis—A symposium. *Calif Med* 114:44, 1971

Wilmot AJ: *Clinical Amoebiasis.* Oxford: Blackwell, 1962

Wolfe MS: Nondysenteric intestinal amebiasis. Treatment with diloxanide furoate. *JAMA* 224:1601, 1973

SUMMARY

Entamoeba histolytica is found throughout the world and is probably the most important parasite causing intestinal symptoms, especially diarrhea. In its invasive phase, the organism penetrates the mucosa of the large intestine, causing abscesses that open into the lumen and form ulcers. These may grow large and be followed by bacterial invasion. Perforation and peritonitis may follow. The large ulcers are due to coalescence of small ones, most typically having the form of "collar buttons." The organism often lives as a commensal. Therefore, the presence of its cysts in the stool is not proof that it is the etiologic agent of the disease.

There are five clinical forms of the disease. Acute ulcerative proctocolitis produces mucosanguineous stools, colicky low abdominal pain, and tenesmus. The diagnosis is based on proctosigmoidoscopic findings and identification of *E. histolytica* in fresh stools. The condition must be differentiated from Crohn's disease, ischemic proctocolitis, acute *Shigella* colitis, and schistosomiasis.

Fulminating colitis presents the same symptoms as ulcerative amebiasis, plus high fever, tachycardia, and hypotension. The abdomen is tender with at times signs of acute peritonitis. The laboratory work-up and flat film of the abdomen show typical findings. Proctoscopy must be done very carefully and reveals extensive amebic ulcers.

Amebic typhloappendicitis presents pathology in the cecum and appendix. It is difficult to differentiate from acute appendicitis. When the onset is gradual, amebae in the stool warrant a therapeutic test.

Ameboma is an inflammatory swelling of the colonic mucosa and submucosa, often confused with tumors and proliferative tuberculosis. The diagnosis is made by microscopic examination of tissue.

Chronic amebic colitis is often diagnosed incorrectly in patients with chronic symptoms in whose stools *E. histolytica* cysts are found. Here an attempt should be made to find actual amebic lesions. If these are not present, seek other etiology. Without lesions, these patients may simply be carriers. Asymptomatic patients passing cysts should be treated with diloxanide furoate. Where the condition is invasive, the treatment is metronidazole. In each instance, alcohol must be forbidden. Emetine or dehydroemetine IM may also be used, but not in patients with cardiopathy.

Giardiasis

31

Trophozoites and cysts of *Giardia lamblia* are frequently found in the duodenum and stools. Statistics indicate an incidence of 2 to 25 per cent in the world's population. Areas of increased risk of infestation include the Soviet Union, South and Southeast Asia, West and Central Africa, Mexico, Korea, and western South America. Endemicity in the United States is low, but in recent years several large-scale outbreaks, which were usually related to contaminated water supplies, have been reported.

Many people infested with *G. lamblia* suffer no digestive symptoms. This fact, and the opinion held formerly that the organism lacked invasive power, explains why *G. lamblia* was considered nonpathogenic. We now know that the parasite can invade the intestinal mucosa. Microscopic and ultramicroscopic studies have proved this. It's also clear that *G. lamblia* can cause various symptoms, especially diarrhea: sometimes acute but mild diarrhea of short duration; at other times severe, especially in children. Some patients may have chronic intestinal symptoms with intermittent diarrhea and flatulence. Foul stools associated with increased flatus and abdominal distention are more characteristic of giardiasis than of other acute diarrheal diseases. Other patients suffer from dyspepsia and epigastric pain, probably from duodenitis caused by the parasite. This pain is very similar to that of peptic ulcer and can be confused with it.

Sometimes *G. lamblia* is associated with a malabsorption syndrome. In these cases hypogammaglobulinemia, especially affecting IgA and IgM levels, often occurs, as well as nodular lymphoid hyperplasia of the small intestine, which may be seen by X-ray.

Although we don't know why clinical symptoms vary so in *G. lamblia* infestation, we can suppose that the number and virulence of the organisms, the host's nutritional state and age, and the concomitant presence of enteropathogenic bacteria have much to do with them. Neither do we understand why the parasite sometimes causes a malabsorption syndrome. Numerous theories have been advanced, such as damage to the intestinal epithelium, a mechanical barrier formed by the parasites that covers the intestinal wall in massive infestation, changes in intestinal mobility, competition for food between the parasite and the host, and antifolic acid effect. Perhaps the explanation lies in a combination of several or all of the factors mentioned, which may vary from patient to patient.

Another unsolved problem concerns the relationship between *G. lamblia* and hypogammaglobulinemia. Sometimes eradication of the parasite not only alleviates symptoms but restores the immunoglobulins to normal. This would suggest that the hypogammaglobulinemia could be secondary to the infestation. But in other patients, perhaps the majority, hypogammaglobulinemia persists. The hypogammaglobulinemia in these cases is probably primary; the association with *G. lamblia* and lymphoid hyperplasia of the small intestine is unexplained.

The diagnosis of infestation with *G. lamblia* is usually made by stool examination. Many stools may be negative in spite of the presence of the parasite in the duodenum. This is proved by finding *G. lamblia* in the duodenal fluid. The duodenal mucus is aspirated through the peroral tube used in taking small intestinal biopsies. Biopsies of the intestinal mucosa may show the parasite as well as shortening and thickening of the villi, chronic or acute inflammation, increased epithelial mitosis, cellular damage, and lymphoid hyperplasia. Some workers have reported the Enterotest, a gelatin capsule containing a string, to be effective in recovering parasites from the duodenum.

In all cases of diarrhea, and especially in patients with unexplained malabsorption syndrome, a thorough search should be made for *G. lamblia.* Failure to find the parasite in the presence of a high index of suspicion justifies a therapeutic trial.

Quinacrine (Atabrine, Atebrin) has been effectively used in eradicating the parasite. One hundred milligrams three times a day for seven days is the dose in adults. Chronic cases may be resistant to treatment, and recurrences are common. A drug equal in effectiveness to quinacrine is metronidazole, 250 mg three times a day for 10 days. This is very effective. Furazolidone (Furoxone), which is available as a suspension, is particularly useful in young children.

Bibliography

Brandenborg LL, Tankersley CB, Gottlieb S, et al: Histologic demonstration of mucosal invasion by Giardia lamblia in man. *Gastroenterology* 52:143, 1967

Wolfe MS: Current concepts in parasitology. Giardiasis. *N Engl J Med* 298:319, 1978

SUMMARY

Many persons with *Giardia lamblia* are symptom-free but may have diarrhea associated with other gastrointestinal symptoms. At times, the organism is associated with a malabsorption syndrome. Usually here hypogammaglobulinemia is present and may be the primary condition. Diagnosis is made via stool examination. If negative, the organism may be found in duodenal fluid obtained by aspiration and/or biopsy of the intestinal mucosa. Treatment is quinacrine (Atabrine, Atebrin), metronidazole (Flagyl), or furazolidone (Furoxone), which is very effective in children.

Intestinal helminthiasis

32

Helminths found frequently in
North America are listed in Table
32-1.

The epidemiologic importance of the intestinal helminths
is enormous. But as causes of diarrhea, they pale beside
pathogenic viruses, bacteria, and amebae. Infestation with
helminths is common. Often they cause no symptoms or
only mild, intermittent diarrhea accompanied by other digestive symptoms such as abdominal pain, meteorism, nausea, and vomiting as well as systemic symptoms such as anorexia, malaise, pallor, headache, urticaria, and weight
loss. A physician practicing where sanitation is good does
not find these parasites of great clinical importance. Where

TABLE 32-1

Helminths found frequently in North America

1. *Taenia*	5. *Trichocephalus*
T. saginata	*Trichuris trichiura*
T. solium	6. *Ascaris*
2. *Diphyllobothrium latum*	*A. lumbricoides*
3. *Hymenolepis*	7. *Uncinaria*
H. nana	*Ancylostoma duodenale*
H. diminuta	*Necator americanus*
4. *Enterobius*	8. *Strongyloides*
E. vermicularis	*S. stercoralis*

sanitation is poor, however, they may cause symptoms that are severe and even life-threatening. For instance, *Trichuris* is asymptomatic when there are fewer than 1,000 eggs/gm of feces; when the infestation is massive, more than 5,000 eggs/gm, it causes important colonic symptoms: diarrhea, dysentery, and anemia. This happens with the majority of intestinal helminths, especially *Hymenolepis; Ascaris,* whose surgical complications are well known (intestinal obstruction); *Necator* and *Ancylostoma,* which cause the greatest pathology; and *Strongyloides.*

The clinician taking care of patients who have lived in areas of the world where intestinal parasites are prevalent must, in all cases of acute or chronic diarrhea, consider the possibility of infestation with helminths and order the indicated laboratory tests.

Bibliography

Markell EK, Voge M: *Medical Parasitology,* 4th ed. Philadelphia: Saunders, 1976

Marsden PD, Schultz MG: Intestinal parasites. *Gastroenterology* 57:724, 1969

Tourist diarrhea

33

The 20th century, with all of its amazing technologic advances, especially in transportation, has created a new member of the human fauna: the tourist. And this tourist can count on an inseparable companion in his gastronomic adventures: diarrhea. This acute, violent, but transient illness of a few days' duration does not seriously interfere with pleasures of sightseeing and is usually quickly forgotten. Sometimes, however, this diarrhea may become serious because of hydroelectrolytic imbalances, toxicity, and other complications.

Tourist diarrhea, called also *turista*, Montezuma's revenge, Aztec two-step, or Delhi belly, has become the subject of many jokes. The fear of this illness discourages some people from venturing away from home. On the other hand, much scientific research has been done on this worldwide problem. Tourist diarrhea can affect any traveler in any part of the world. The clinical picture does not differ from the acute diarrheas that affect native populations. The frequency of tourist diarrhea is proportional to the frequency of diarrhea in the place he visits, since its etiology depends on the same factors that cause diarrhea in the inhabitants of that region. The only difference is that the tourist suffers more frequently because of lack of resistance to endemic organisms.

Like native inhabitants, tourists suffer from acute diarrhea as a result of dietary indiscretions, food spoilage, excess alcohol intake, and, occasionally, enteric infections and infestations. Bacteria (*Shigella, Salmonella, Escherichia coli*), protozoa (*Entamoeba histolytica* and *Giardia lamblia*), and possibly helminths and viruses may be responsible. Prospective and retrospective studies have confirmed this multiplicity of causes.

One outstanding discovery has been the isolation of *E. coli* strains that until recently had not been considered pathogenic from stools of patients with tourist diarrhea. As we now know, the organism has invasive tendencies or the ability to produce toxins which, like the cholera vibrio's, stimulate the intestine to secrete enormous amounts of water and electrolytes. The pathogenicity of these strains of *E. coli* is no longer in doubt, and these organisms are accepted as the most frequent cause of tourist diarrhea. On the other hand, these strains of *E. coli* rarely cause diarrhea in adult permanent residents, probably because an ecologic equilibrium has been arrived at through the hosts' immunologic defenses. This view is supported by the fact that *E. coli* strains cause acute infectious diarrhea in small children, whose immunologic defenses are still immature. Tourists coming from less contaminated areas apparently lack the corresponding antibodies.

Treatment of tourist diarrhea is quite simple and should be limited to a 24-hour fast, allowing only clear liquids, as well as symptomatic treatment with mild antispasmodics

and antidiarrheal agents (belladonna alkaloids, diphenoxylate, loperamide, kaolin, pectin, and, sometimes, paregoric elixir). It is unwise to stop the diarrhea entirely and
prematurely, thus interfering with a defense mechanism.
Antidiarrheal agents should be used sparingly, with the
sole purpose of decreasing the severity of the diarrhea.
   Culture of the stool and examination for trophozoites of
amebae and *Giardia,* and specific treatment of these organisms if they are found, is always recommended. Antibiotics
are generally unnecessary. They're even contraindicated in
Salmonella infections and are of doubtful benefit in
shigellosis and *E. coli* infections. These are self-limited illnesses, and the antibiotics' undesirable effects probably out-
weigh their value. They should be reserved for severe cases
in which toxicity and bacteremia make them necessary.
Hospitalization, oral and parenteral fluids, glucose, and
electrolytes may be required in cases of dehydration and
electrolyte imbalance.
   Very little has been proved scientifically regarding prophylaxis. Studies without adequate controls indicate the
possible benefit of nonabsorbable sulfa drugs and neomycin.
However, because of the potential toxicity and doubtful
value of these drugs, their use should not be recommended.
The best prophylaxis is prudence and moderation in eating
and drinking.
   Mention should be made, however, of a double-blind study
of Peace Corps volunteers in Kenya which proved that
doxycycline (one 100-mg capsule daily with breakfast) effectively prevented most episodes of traveler's diarrhea.

Bibliography

Gorbach SL, Kean BH, Evans DG, et al: Traveler's diarrhea and toxigenic
   Escherichia coli. *N Engl J Med* 292:933, 1975

Merson MH, Gangarosa EJ: Traveler's diarrhea. *JAMA* 234:200, 1975

Merson MH, Morris GK, Sack DA, et al: Traveler's diarrhea in Mexico: A
   prospective study of physicians and family members attending a congress. *N Engl J Med* 294:1299, 1976

Sack DA, Kaminsky DC, Sack RB, et al: Prophylactic doxycycline for trav-
   eller's diarrhea. *N Engl J Med* 298:758, 1978

SUMMARY

Tourist diarrhea occurs all over the world and doesn't differ from the diarrhea of native populations, although tourists suffer more frequently because of lack of resistance to the prevailing organisms. This diarrhea results from dietary indiscretion, food spoilage, excess alcohol, bacterial or protozoan infections, and possibly worms and viruses. The most frequent cause is *E. coli* enteropathogen. Treatment consists of a 24-hour fast with only clear liquids permitted, mild antispasmodics, and antidiarrheals. Antibiotics are usually not indicated except in severe cases. Recently, in Kenya, it was shown that 100 mg doxycycline with breakfast was a good preventative.

Pseudo-membranous enterocolitis

34

Pseudomembranous enterocolitis is a syndrome resulting from several causes and combining a group of pathologic lesions and clinical symptoms and signs.

The lesions are located in the colon and/or small intestine. They consist of multiple yellow membranous plaques varying in size from 3 to 20 mm. When they coalesce, they form a sheet resembling the false membrane of diphtheria. The intervening mucosa is hyperemic. Underneath the plaques the mucosa is edematous, friable, congested, or even dotted with superficial ulcerations. The membranes are made up of fibrin, mucus, necrotic cells, polymorphonuclear leukocytes, and bacteria. The epithelium shows areas of necrosis, erosions, and inflammatory, purulent exudate, as does the lamina propria. The submucosa is frankly congested and edematous. In the most severe cases, true gangrene of the epithelium uncovers ulcers of various sizes.

The clinical picture is characterized by more-or-less sudden onset of diarrhea in patients who are already seriously ill. The stools are very frequent, large, and liquid and contain mucus, pus, and, rarely, fresh blood. The patient has fever and looks toxic. Dehydration, electrolyte imbalance, acidosis, and shock quickly develop. The primary illnesses in which this alarming complication develops are intestinal obstruction, cardiac disease, shock, renal insufficiency, and postoperative states, especially following abdominal surgery. Ischemia of the bowel seems to be the common denominator.

The clinical picture varies, depending on whether the syndrome appears as a primary severe disease or is associated with antibiotics. Diarrhea is a frequent complication of antibiotic therapy. In most cases the only proctoscopic findings are edema and nonspecific granularity. The development of pseudomembranous enterocolitis in patients receiving broad-spectrum antibiotics has been documented but, until recently, was considered rare. Nevertheless, two antibiotics, clindamycin (Cleocin) and the closely related lincomycin (Lincocin), have been reported to cause this syndrome in up to 10 per cent of patients receiving them. The disturbance is due to the effect of toxins of *Clostridium difficile.* In some instances the syndrome is associated with recovery of *Staphylococcus aureus* from intestinal contents, but the exact relationship of this organism to the disease is not clearly defined. The onset may be gradual or abrupt, with fever from 38° to 40°C associated with watery diarrhea and cramps. The stools may contain mucus, pus, and, on occasion, blood. The majority of cases reported have been of moderate severity, although the diarrhea was frequent (up to 30 stools per day), leading to dehydration and metabolic acidosis. The diarrhea may begin to subside in the first week but usually lasts two to three weeks or longer. Abdominal distention occurs and is sometimes accompanied by toxic dilation of the colon.

The diagnosis of pseudomembranous enterocolitis should be suspected when a fulminating toxic diarrhea develops as a complication of one of the severe diseases previously listed or when it appears in a patient receiving antibiotics, particularly clindamycin or lincomycin. Under any of these circumstances, sigmoidoscopy should be all that is necessary to establish the correct diagnosis. No other disease is characterized by the raised, yellowish plaques on an erythematous base. X-rays may be helpful but rarely are necessary. Plain films show markedly edematous haustral markings and an increase in the overall thickness of the colonic wall. The stool may reveal clusters of gram-positive cocci, suggesting *S. aureus*. Culture of stool or exudate will yield *Cl. difficile*.

Treatment is concerned first with vigorous measures to prevent or combat shock and electrolyte imbalance, such as blood, plasma, plasma proteins, water, electrolytes, pressor agents, and steroids. As in enterotoxic diarrhea, enormous amounts of liquids may be required: 10 to 15 liters in 24 hours. If large clusters of staphylococci are seen on fecal smear, methicillin (Staphcillin), cephalothin (Keflin), or erythromycin should be administered. If pseudomembranous enterocolitis began while the patient was taking an antimicrobial drug, the medication must be withdrawn and vancomycin (Vancocin), 0.5 gm intravenously twice daily, must be given while the results of the stool culture are awaited.

Bibliography

Alpers DH: The pseudomembranous enterocolitides. In *Gastrointestinal Disease* (Sleisenger MH, Fordtran JS, eds), 2nd ed, p 1715. Philadelphia: Saunders, 1978

Bartlett JG, Moon N, Chang TW, et al: Role of Clostridium difficile in antibiotic-associated pseudomembranous colitis. *Gastroenterology* 75:778, 1978

Tedesco FJ: Clindamycin-associated colitis. A review of the clinical spectrum of 47 cases. *Am J Dig Dis* 21:26, 1976

SUMMARY

When a fulminating, toxic diarrhea complicates intestinal obstruction, cardiac disease, shock, renal insufficiency, postoperative states, especially recovery from abdominal surgery, or antibiotic therapy, the diagnosis of pseudomembranous enterocolitis should be suspected. Sigmoidoscopy reveals the pathognomonic raised yellow plaques on an erythematous base. The clinical picture is sudden onset of diarrhea with frequent large, liquid stools containing mucus and pus and at times blood, with fever, dehydration, electrolyte imbalance, acidosis, and shock. Treatment is aimed at combating shock and electrolyte imbalance. If there are many staphylococci in the stool, methicillin (Staphcillin), cephalothin (Keflin), or erythromycin should be given. If the disease follows antibiotic therapy, the drug must be withdrawn and IV vancomycin (Vancocin) introduced until stool culture results are in.

Chronic nonspecific ulcerative colitis

35

Chronic nonspecific ulcerative colitis is an inflammatory disease of the colon. Of unknown etiology, it affects the rectum and colon. The damage characteristically involves the mucosal and submucosal layers with vascular congestion, hemorrhage, ulcerations, atrophy, pseudopolyps, and narrowing of the intestinal lumen. In contrast to other types of colitis, where the lesions are discrete, the damage here is diffuse and continuous. The terminal part of the ileum may be involved. Unlike granulomatous colitis, chronic ulcerative colitis does not cause fistulae or leave areas of mucosa free of inflammation. Microscopically there is mucosal and submucosal infiltration with polymorphonuclear leukocytes, lymphocytes, plasma cells, and eosinophils. Crypt abscesses, hemorrhages, and ulcers occur frequently. No granulomas, intramural sinuses, or significant submucosal fibrosis are present, but loss of mucosal epithelium is characteristic of the disease.

Clinical picture

The disease tends to occur between the second and fourth decades of life and is more common in women and Caucasians, especially Jews. Its severity, evolution, and prognosis vary greatly. Its onset may be gradual or sudden. Main symptoms are intestinal bleeding, diarrhea, abdominal pain, fever, and loss of weight. Its progress may be intermittent, recurrences alternating with remissions. Only a few have a continuous, progressive form with no remissions.

Clinicians are agreed in classifying chronic nonspecific ulcerative colitis into three types: mild, moderate, and severe or fulminant. The mild form, also called ulcerative proctitis, is the most common. Only the distal segments of the colon are affected. The symptoms are tenesmus, diarrhea, and slight rectal bleeding. Systemic symptoms are absent. In the moderate form, diarrhea is the outstanding symptom, with a daily average of four to six liquid stools. They contain some mucus and blood and are preceded by colicky pain and followed by tenesmus. Mild fever, anorexia, fatigue, and weight loss accompany the diarrhea. The severe form is rare. Its onset is nearly always sudden, with profuse diarrhea, rectal bleeding, and high fever, either continuous or spiking, tenesmus, and systemic toxicity. The patient looks dehydrated and toxic and may be acidotic and in shock. The abdomen is distended and tender to palpation with signs of peritoneal irritation. The leukocyte count is high, with a shift to the left, and there is anemia and hypoalbuminemia.

Diagnosis

Patients may complain of diarrhea with or without blood, or of rectal bleeding with or without diarrhea. These symptoms point to the presence of colorectal inflammatory or neoplastic disease. Definite diagnosis is established by taking the steps outlined in Part I of this book: anorectal examination, proctosigmoidoscopy, X-ray studies, search for parasites in the stools, and stool cultures. This orderly sequence of studies is indispensable. Anorectal examination rules out fissures, hemorrhoids, polyps, and cancer of the rectum. The proctosigmoidoscopic picture is characteristic and can be considered the key to the diagnosis, though it is not pathognomonic. Shigellosis and sometimes amebiasis may produce the same picture. X-rays support the diagnosis and determine the extent of the process as well as the presence of complications. X-rays may be normal in early and benign forms. Biopsy of the rectal mucosa is unnecessary in typical cases of chronic nonspecific ulcerative colitis but is indicated when sigmoidoscopy is equivocal in the early and benign forms and when it is difficult to rule out amebiasis. In the early and benign forms, biopsy reveals inflammatory changes in the mucosa and crypt abscesses, a finding that many pathologists consider of great diagnostic value. In the case of confusion with amebiasis, the biopsy may reveal vegetative forms of amebae invading the mucosa.

A rather infrequent clinical picture that may be confused with chronic ulcerative colitis is ischemic colitis, which is caused by vascular obstruction in patients with arteriosclerosis. Symptoms of ischemic colitis are abdominal pain of sudden onset, rectal bleeding, vomiting, fever, and signs of peritoneal irritation. Endoscopic findings resemble those of chronic ulcerative colitis, and barium enema shows suggestive changes, such as irregular sawtooth outlines, nodular markings, thumbprinting, sacculations, and narrowing. Ischemic colitis lasts a short time. In severe cases, surgical removal of the ischemic segment is necessary. Mild forms may go on for days and improve spontaneously, often leaving an area of stenosis in the intestine.

Differential diagnosis of chronic ulcerative colitis also includes diverticular disease of the colon, regional enteritis, and especially granulomatous colitis and pseudomembranous colitis. The differential diagnosis should not be difficult except in the case of granulomatous colitis, which markedly resembles chronic ulcerative disease clinically

TABLE 35-1

Anatomic and pathologic differences between ulcerative and granulomatous colitis

Characteristic	Ulcerative colitis	Granulomatous colitis
Distribution	Diffuse, mucosal	Focal, transmural
Intestinal wall	Shortened, without haustra or thickening	Thickened, rigid, edematous, fibrous
Granulomas	Absent	In more than 50%
Crypt abscesses	Frequent	Not frequent
Lymphoid aggregates	Absent	Very frequent
Fissures and tracts	Absent	Very frequent
Anal lesions	15%	85%
Rectal biopsy	Nonspecific inflammation	Noncaseous granulomas

and on biopsy. For this reason many clinicians and researchers maintain that there is no fundamental difference between the two and that there are many intermediate pathologic pictures linking them. Tables 35-1 and 35-2 summarize the principal histologic and clinical differences between ulcerative and granulomatous colitis.

Complications

Complications of chronic nonspecific ulcerative colitis are many, and some are serious (Table 35-3). Anorectal complications are not as common as in granulomatous colitis. The pseudopolyps are islands of normal mucosa or granulation tissue surrounded by ulcers. Neither one is a premalignant lesion, as was formerly supposed.

Toxic megacolon is a very serious complication of chronic ulcerative colitis as well as of granulomatous and amebic ulcerative colitis, although less frequent in these two latter diseases. It seems to result from extension of the inflammatory process from the mucosa and submucosa, where it ordinarily stops, to the muscular coat. Opium derivatives, diphenoxylate and atropine (Lomotil), and anticholinergics

TABLE 35-2

Clinical differences between granulomatous and ulcerative colitis

Change	Granulomatous colitis	Ulcerative colitis
Intestinal		
Rectal hemorrhage	Rare	Frequent
Sigmoidoscopy	Normal or discrete lesions	Abnormal, diffuse lesions
Fistulae	Frequent	No
Perianal disease	Frequent	Rare
Abdominal pain	Frequent	Rare
Abdominal mass	Frequent	No
Stenosis	Frequent	Rare
Distribution of lesions	Discontinuous; entire digestive tract	Continuous; rectum and colon
Frequency of cancer	Increased	Very much increased
Extraintestinal		
Arthritis	Occasional	Occasional
Dermatitis	Occasional	Occasional
Iritis and episcleritis	Occasional	Occasional
Hydronephrosis	Occasional	No
Liver pathology	Occasional	Occasional
Systemic		
Amyloidosis	Increased frequency	Rare
Anemia	Frequent	Frequent
Fever	Frequent	Frequent
Cholelithiasis	Increased frequency	Normal frequency
Retarded growth	Frequent	Frequent
Kidney stones	Occasional	Occasional

in high doses may be responsible. The abdomen suddenly becomes greatly distended and painful; signs of peritoneal reaction occur (pain on compression and decompression, absence of peristaltic sounds, tympany) as well as high fever, tachycardia, and prostration. A plain film of the abdomen shows marked dilation of all or part of the colon with irregular, raveled mucosa whose edges are sawtoothed. Proctosig-

TABLE 35-3

Complications of nonspecific chronic ulcerative colitis

Local	Systemic
Hemorrhoids, anal fissures, anal fistulae, perianal abscess, ischiorectal abscess, rectal prolapse, rectovaginal fistula Pseudopolyps Toxic megacolon Perforation of the colon Cancer of the colon Stenosis of the colon Massive hemorrhage	Hepatic disease: pericholangitis, sclerosing cholangitis, chronic active hepatitis, cirrhosis Joint disease Ocular lesions: uveitis Skin lesions: pyoderma gangrenosum

moidoscopy shows ulcerative colitis. This finding is of great importance in cases where the past history is unknown. These symptoms could lead to an erroneous diagnosis of acute abdomen.

Medical treatment of toxic megacolon consists of nasogastric suction, parenteral solutions, and ACTH (40 to 60 units) or prednisolone (100 to 200 mg) by intravenous drip. If there is no improvement in two or three days, surgery should be performed because of the danger of perforation. Decompression with ileostomy, cecostomy, or, less often, subtotal colectomy is the surgical treatment.

Cancer of the colon is 10 times as frequent in patients with chronic ulcerative colitis as in the general population and its frequency is in direct proportion to the disease's duration, extent, and continuous progress without remissions. The risk is increased when the disease begins before 21 years of age and when it has lasted more than 10 years.

Stenosis of the colon from scarring may be confused with neoplasm. In spite of the benign nature of chronic ulcerative colitis, surgery may be justified. Severe hemorrhages are rare and stop spontaneously. Treatment is blood transfusions, ACTH, and close observation of the patient until the hemorrhage stops.

Hepatic complications are pericholangitis, steatosis, chronic active hepatitis, cirrhosis, and sclerosing cholangitis. Most of these lesions do not improve after the diseased colon has been removed surgically.

Arthritis in patients with chronic ulcerative colitis or other inflammatory diseases of the intestine affects the large and medium-sized joints, is migratory, and resolves without sequelae. Ten per cent of patients with chronic ulcerative colitis develop arthritis. Joint symptoms coincide with exacerbations of the intestinal disease. Ankylosing spondylitis is especially common. These patients belong to a definite genotype with histocompatibility antigen HLA-B27. This supports the hypothesis that genetic factors are important in the pathogenicity of this disease.

Iritis, erythema nodosum, and pyoderma gangrenosum are other complications. Their presence should point to the diagnosis of chronic ulcerative colitis.

Psychological management

The management of patients with nonspecific chronic ulcerative colitis is complex. Since its etiology is unknown, there is no specific treatment. Its tendency to affect people who are psychologically abnormal makes therapy difficult and influences the course of the disease. Many patients with chronic ulcerative colitis are immature, rigid, hypersensitive, and dependent on a key figure (usually the mother). Whether these traits are primary or secondary to a chronic debilitating disease has not been settled. However, it's known that emotional factors play an important role in the exacerbations and remissions of the disease and that the physician's human qualities are at least as important as the pharmacologic tools he applies in determining the outcome of his therapeutic intervention.

Treatment

Since nonspecific ulcerative colitis is a chronic relapsing disease, it's necessary to consider the treatment of the acute stages as well as the prevention of relapses. Treatment of the benign form is relatively simple. The diet should be low in residues. Clinical and laboratory tests should be done to determine whether the patient tolerates lactose. If not, milk should be omitted from the diet.

Sulfasalazine

Sulfasalazine (Azulfidine) sparked controversy for several years. Some clinicians insisted the drug was superior to any other sulfa or antibiotic, while others maintained it had no more value than a placebo. Strictly controlled studies, done recently, have established the drug's value. The recommended dose is 0.5 to 1 gm every four hours during the active stage of colitis. Some workers state that it not only shortens the acute stage but also helps to prevent relapses. They recommend its daily use for periods as long as a year or more. Sulfasalazine consists of sulfapyridine linked by an azo bond to 5-aminosalicylic acid. Bacterial cleavage of this bond appears essential for optimal therapeutic effectiveness. The observation that 5-aminosalicylic acid inhibits mucosal prostaglandin synthetase activity, thereby reducing tissue prostaglandin levels, provides an important insight into the pathophysiology of colitis. Sulfasalazine is not always well tolerated; more than a third of patients have anorexia, nausea, vomiting, dizziness, and headache. A small number have serious reactions, such as dermatosis, fever, and blood dyscrasias.

Steroids

Corticosteroids are of great value in treating nonspecific ulcerative colitis. They usually produce rapid remission. Some favor prednisone, 40 mg/day, but other corticosteroids in equivalent doses are also effective. As soon as a clinical remission takes place, the dose may be gradually reduced and, if possible, the drug discontinued.

Many clinicians prefer ACTH, 20 to 40 units/day in normal saline or 5 per cent glucose intravenously over eight hours. No satisfactory studies have shown the superiority of ACTH. In benign forms of disease, corticosteroids are often given by rectum in the form of suppositories or enemas, especially if the lesions are in the rectum and distal colon. Results are excellent in most cases. The suppositories contain 10 mg of cortisol (hydrocortisone) or 5 to 10 mg of prednisone 11-phosphate. Retention enemas contain 100 to 200 mg of hydrocortisone acetate, 10 mg of prednisone, or 40 mg of methylprednisolone acetate dissolved in 150 ml or less of normal saline, given at night. If the patient has trouble retaining the enema, 30 mg of codeine can be given half an hour before.

Some clinicians disapprove of the use of corticosteroids, especially in the benign form of chronic ulcerative colitis. However, they are useful because they promptly control symptoms; this helps establish confidence in the physician. The dosage should be reduced gradually and the drug withdrawn as soon as warranted in order to avoid or attenuate its side effects.

Symptomatic treatment of the diarrhea is diphenoxylate and atropine in low doses with hydrophilic colloids.

Treatment of acute stages

If the patient has a serious attack of ulcerative colitis, he should be hospitalized and treated with corticosteroids—ACTH, prednisone, or other preparations. The dose should be moderately high—40 units of ACTH or 40 to 60 mg of prednisone—until there is definite improvement, at which time it can be gradually and carefully reduced. ACTH can be changed to prednisone after five to 10 days. Azulfidine should be given at the same time, 1 gm every four hours, and continued for a long period since it may prevent relapses. Diet should be low in residues, preferably without milk or milk products until it is clear that the patient can tolerate these foods. In these severe forms of ulcerative colitis, anemia and fluid and electrolyte imbalance may occur suddenly. These must be promptly treated with blood transfusions and intravenous solutions. Loss of potassium is frequent and should be immediately corrected.

Fulminating ulcerative colitis is a true medical emergency. The mortality is high, either from acute toxic dilation of the colon or from perforation and peritonitis. The patient should be hospitalized at once and given ACTH as described above. If there is no distention, clear fluids may be taken by mouth; but if there is distention, gastric suction must be started. It is very important to check and control body fluid and electrolyte levels and to correct anemia and protein loss with blood transfusions and albumin, respectively. An antibiotic should be given, preferably ampicillin.

The patient must be closely watched by both the internist and surgeon. Parenteral hyperalimentation is very helpful in these cases, giving the colon a physiological rest (Appendix F). If there is any suspicion of perforation, from either clinical findings or X-rays, or if the patient is not definitely better in three or four days, an ileostomy and colectomy are in order.

Prevention of relapses

Treatment of nonspecific chronic ulcerative colitis includes not only caring for the patient in the acute stages but also the prevention of relapses. To accomplish this, a low-residue diet must be adhered to and the patient directed to lead a life free from excesses and overexertion. Azulfidine, 2 gm/day for long periods, even a year, may be effective. Some patients need small doses of corticosteroids, 5 to 10 mg of prednisone a day, to prevent relapses. But the most important part of the therapy is a good physician-patient relationship. To some extent the doctor should become the key figure on whom the patient feels he can depend. Encourage such patients to express their hostilities openly so that they can be dealt with in a mature manner, fostering emotional growth. Causing frustrations, failing patients in their expectations, disappointing them with false promises, breaking appointments, leaving town without letting them know who is covering for you—all should be avoided. Care of these individuals is difficult and often taxes the patience. However, your efforts will be rewarded by long periods of remission due more to this relationship than to medication.

Surgery

The surgical treatment of chronic ulcerative colitis consists of total colectomy with permanent ileostomy. This major surgical procedure sacrifices the diseased colon and leaves a problem, the ileostomy. One thing is certain: Removal of the colon cures the disease. When colectomy is really indicated, it rehabilitates chronic invalids who otherwise have no hope of improvement. It even saves lives. Indications for colectomy are (1) serious complications such as toxic megacolon unresponsive to medical treatment, cancer of the colon, perforation, severe uncontrollable hemorrhage, and fistulae, (2) failure of medical treatment as demonstrated by lack of improvement, especially in fulminating forms and toxic megacolon, or losing weight, strength, and ability to carry on a normal life. These patients are much better off with an ileostomy than with ulcerative colitis. For a successful outcome, the surgery must be expertly done and the patient must be prepared psychologically to manage his ileostomy. The Kock reservoir (continent) ileostomy is an effective alternative to conventional ileostomy in ulcerative colitis. Groups of people who have had this operation form clubs and are most helpful to each other psychologically and practically.

Bibliography

Cello JP, Meyer JH: Ulcerative colitis. In *Gastrointestinal Disease* (Sleisenger MH, Fordtran JS, eds), 2nd ed, p 1597. Philadelphia: Saunders, 1978

Dissanyake A, Truelove S: A controlled therapeutic trial of long-term maintenance treatment of ulcerative colitis with sulphasalazine. *Gut* 14:818, 1973

Gear EV Jr, Dobbins WO: Rectal biopsy. A review of its diagnostic usefulness. *Gastroenterology* 55:522, 1968

Klotz U, Maier K, Fischer C, et al: Therapeutic efficacy of sulfasalazine and its metabolites in patients with ulcerative colitis and Crohn's disease. *N Engl J Med* 303:1499, 1980

Kock NS: Intra-abdominal reservoir in patients with permanent ileostomy. Preliminary observations on a procedure resulting in fecal continence in five ileostomy patients. *Arch Surg* 99:223, 1969

Palmer WL, Crane RT: The therapeutic role of corticotropin and corticosteroids in nonspecific inflammatory disease of the intestine. *Ann Intern Med* 58:1063, 1963

Pardo SA, Perez ANG, Zavala B: Colitis crónica inespecifica y colitis ulcerosa amibiana. Diagnóstico diferencial. *Rev Gastroenterol Mex* 36:13, 1971

Turnbull RB Jr, Schofield PF, Hawk WA: Nonspecific ulcerative colitis. *Adv Surg* 3:161, 1968

SUMMARY

Chronic nonspecific ulcerative colitis is an inflammatory disease of the rectum and colon (the terminal part of the ileum may also be involved) of unknown etiology. Vascular congestion, hemorrhage, ulceration, mucosal atrophy, pseudopolyps, and narrowing of the intestinal lumen occur in a diffuse and continuous manner. Onset may be sudden or gradual. The main symptoms are intestinal bleeding, diarrhea, abdominal pain, fever, and weight loss. It tends to be recurrent with periods of remission and is classified as mild, moderate, or severe (fulminant). The symptoms of the mild form are tenesmus, diarrhea, and slight rectal bleeding; of the moderate form, diarrhea of four to six liquid stools per day with mucus and blood preceded by colicky pain and tenesmus, mild fever, anorexia, fatigue, and weight loss; of the severe form (rare), sudden onset with profuse diarrhea, rectal bleeding, high fever, tenesmus, systemic toxicity, abdominal distention, signs of peritoneal irritation, and shock.

Chronic ulcerative colitis must be differentiated from shigellosis, amebiasis, ischemic colitis due to vascular obstruction by arteriosclerosis, diverticular disease of the colon, regional enteritis, granulomatous colitis, and pseudomembranous colitis (see Tables 35-1, 35-2, and 35-3). Toxic megacolon is one of the most serious complications and must be heroically treated, to the point of subtotal colectomy, in order to prevent perforation. Carcinoma of the colon is 10 times more frequent in persons with chronic ulcerative colitis than in the general population. Pericholangitis, steatosis, chronic active hepatitis, cirrhosis, and sclerosing cholangitis are some of the liver complications. Arthritis, particularly ankylosing spondylitis, iritis, erythema nodosum, and pyoderma gangrenosum are other complications.

Treatment is difficult since emotional factors play an important role. In general, however, a low-residue diet, sulfasalazine, corticosteroids or ACTH, and symptomatics for diarrhea are in order. Fluid and electrolyte imbalance must be remedied quickly. Fulminating ulcerative colitis is a medical emergency.

Granulomatous (transmural) colitis

36

Until recently it was thought that Crohn's disease was limited to the small intestine. This is not the case. Many patients diagnosed as having nonspecific ulcerative colitis are actually suffering from Crohn's disease of the colon. The disease has been called "Crohn's disease of the colon," "Crohn's colitis," "granulomatous colitis," "segmental colitis," and, recently, "transmural colitis." The last term seems most appropriate. The pathology is the same as in the small intestine: thickening of the walls, narrowing of the lumen, and fistula formation. Microscopically, deep ulcers and fissures, total involvement of the wall, and noncaseous granulomas are seen. The rectum frequently, but not always, escapes involvement.

When it is involved, biopsy shows granulomas, a finding of considerable diagnostic importance. Usually only non-specific inflammatory changes are seen. The colon is involved in a discontinuous manner, lesions becoming localized in one or more segments. Very frequently the disease involves both the colon and the small intestine. This is the type most commonly seen.

Symptoms are similar to those in any inflammatory and ulcerative disease of the colon: diarrhea, bleeding, low abdominal pain, fever, malaise, and weight loss. Perianal abscesses and fistulas are very common. The diarrhea is of the type seen in colitis: semiliquid or liquid stools, not large, generally without blood although at times large amounts of blood may be present. The desire to defecate is urgent and is preceded by colicky pain in the lower abdomen. Tenesmus is not rare. Eating, exercising, and nervous excitement precipitate the desire to defecate.

Proctosigmoidoscopic examination frequently shows perianal lesions: abscesses, large painless fissures, and fleshy or nodular skin tags. The rectal mucosa may look normal, contrasting markedly with the appearance of nonspecific ulcerative colitis, or it may appear to be moderately congested and granular. Less frequently, it has a cobblestone surface and isolated, irregular ulcers with a whitish base similar to amebic ulcers and separated by normal mucosa (see Chapter 15).

The X-ray abnormalities of granulomatous colitis were described in detail in Chapter 20. Noteworthy characteristics are the isolated lesions, the transverse and linear ulcers and fissures, the lack of symmetry of the intramural lesions, and the fistulae.

Treatment of Crohn's disease of the colon is similar to treatment of the disease when it affects the small intestine. Surgery should be avoided if at all possible because of very frequent relapses. Rest is helpful; hospitalization may be necessary in the acute stages. It's important to maintain good nutrition by means of a balanced diet. High-residue, irritating foods should be avoided only if they cause diarrhea or pain. Individuals vary greatly in their tolerance to such foods, and this is not always related to the severity of the disease. Some patients can eat practically anything, especially during remissions. Others have individual intolerances and idiosyncrasies that must be respected. An intolerance of lactose due to lactase deficiency often occurs.

Symptomatic treatment consists of antispasmodics and antidiarrheals. The presence of abscesses requires antibiotics, such as ampicillin, chloramphenicol, cephalosporins, or gentamicin. Sulfasalazine, prescribed for nonspecific ulcerative colitis, has also been used here, but with less success. Controversy exists about the value of ACTH and corticosteroids. Some clinicians use them routinely and claim that they cause the inflammation to subside and improve patients' appetite and sense of well-being. Others assert that adrenal steroids are not only worthless against Crohn's colitis but also favor the development of perianal fistulae and abscesses. Between these two extremes, the adrenal steroids appear moderately useful and should be used as briefly as possible when other methods are insufficient. Sometimes the inflammation and consequent thickening of the walls will narrow the intestine and give rise to symptoms of occlusion. This process improves with intestinal intubation and corticosteroids, saving the patient from surgical intervention. The doses are similar to those used in Crohn's disease of the small intestine and in nonspecific ulcerative colitis. Immunosuppressive agents (azathioprine, 6-mercaptopurine) have been tried, with promising results in some cases.

Surgery should be avoided if possible, because of the marked tendency to relapse so characteristic of Crohn's disease. Relapse happens in at least 50 per cent of patients, and the rate increased to 90 per cent in postoperative patients followed for many years. Recent studies suggest that the ultimate outcomes after proctocolectomy in Crohn's disease of the colon and ulcerative colitis are similar. Sometimes surgery is unavoidable, as in acute or chronic intestinal obstruction unaffected by corticosteroids; persistent severe perianal involvement; formation of fistulae and abscesses; and diarrhea, abdominal pain, fever, and general debility that are refractory to the conservative treatment just outlined. The most common operations are hemicolectomy with anastomosis of the ileum to the transverse colon, segmental resection in other localized forms of the disease, and, when the entire colon is involved, total or subtotal colectomy with ileostomy.

Bibliography

Brooke BN: Granulomatous diseases of the intestine. *Lancet* 2:745, 1959

Fawaz KA, Glotzer DG, Goldman H, et al: Ulcerative colitis and Crohn's disease of the colon—A comparison of the long-term postoperative courses. *Gastroenterology* 71:372, 1976

Lennard-Jones JE, Lockhart-Mummery HE, Morson BC: Clinical and pathological differentiation of Crohn's disease and proctocolitis. *Gastroenterology* 54:1162, 1968

Lindner AE, Marshak RH, Wolf BS, et al: Granulomatous colitis: A clinical study. *N Engl J Med* 269:379, 1963

Lockhart-Mummery HE, Morson BC: Crohn's disease of the large intestine. *Gut* 5:493, 1964

Marshak RH, Lindner AE: *Radiology of the Small Intestine,* 2nd ed. Philadelphia: Saunders, 1976

Present DH, Korelitz BI, Wisch N, et al: Treatment of Crohn's disease with 6-mercaptopurine. *N Engl J Med* 302:981, 1980

Spiro HH: Crohn's colitis. In *Clinical Gastroenterology* (Spiro HH, ed), p 402. London: Macmillan, 1970

Summers RW, Switz DM, Sessions JT, et al: National Cooperative Crohn's Disease Study: Results of drug treatment. *Gastroenterology* 77(pt 2):847, 1978

Zetzell L: Granulomatous (ileo)colitis. *N Engl J Med* 282:600, 1970

SUMMARY

Transmural colitis, another name for granulomatous colitis or Crohn's disease, seems the most appropriate name for this condition. Most commonly, both the small intestine and colon are involved with thickening of the walls, narrowing of the lumen, and fistula formation. The rectum is rarely involved; when it is, the biopsy shows granulomas. The colon is involved sequentially in a discontinuous manner. Symptoms are typical of inflammatory and ulcerative colonic disease. Perianal abscesses and fistulae are common. Treatment consists of rest and hospitalization in the acute phase, maintenance of nutritional status, and attention to food intolerance. Symptomatic treatment with antispasmodics and antidiarrheals may be necessary, and antibiotics if abscesses are present. Some advocate corticosteroids and/or ACTH. Surgery should be avoided because of frequent relapses.

Tumors of the colon and rectum

Benign tumors: Villous adenoma

37

Diarrhea is not an important symptom in patients with benign tumors of the colon and rectum. Many are asymptomatic. Some may notice that their stools have streaks of blood, and a few complain of colicky pain and short spells of mild diarrhea.

This does not hold for the villous (papillary) adenoma. It constitutes only 2 to 14 per cent of polyps of the rectum and colon. It is sessile, with a wide base that merges gradually into the surrounding normal mucosa. Its surface is soft, gelatinous, irregular, papillary, and velvety, with fronds. It produces large amounts of mucus.

The clinical significance of the villous adenoma is its greater tendency to become malignant than other adenomas, and the large quantities of mucus, water, and electrolytes it secretes. Normal stools contain up to 5 mEq of sodium and 15 mEq of potassium in 24 hours. Villous adenomas may secrete daily 160 mEq of sodium and 80 mEq of potassium. If the adenoma occurs in the cecum or ascending colon, the distal part of the large bowel can reabsorb a large part of these fluids and electrolytes and restore them to the extracellular spaces, but if the tumor is in the distal part of the colon or in the rectum, nothing prevents the loss and the consequent dehydration, hyponatremia, and hypokalemia.

At first the tumor secretes small amounts of mucus that are eliminated mixed with feces. As the tumor becomes larger, mucus production increases and finally causes severe, watery diarrhea with 15 to 20 stools in 24 hours, accompanied by hyponatremia and hypokalemia as well as by hypotonic dehydration.

Suspect a villous adenoma as the cause of the diarrhea when there is much mucus or when the diarrhea resists treatment with nonspecific antidiarrheals and is accompanied by hypokalemia. Some patients complain of mucous discharge from the anus severe enough to require wearing diapers, although their stools may be solid.

Diagnosis is usually made by rectal palpation followed by proctosigmoidoscopic examination and biopsy. If the tumor is high up, barium enema and colonoscopy with biopsy should give the necessary information. Chapter 15 describes the problems of identifying villous adenomas.

Treatment is removal of the tumor. If histologic examination reveals malignant changes, and especially if there has been tissue invasion, radical surgery is indicated.

Malignant tumors
of the colon and rectum

The division of malignant tumors of the colon into those of the right colon and those of the left colon is classical. Those of the right colon cause anemia and a palpable mass; those of the left colon cause rectal bleeding and symptoms of obstruction. Diarrhea is not important in either. It occurs occasionally but gives no important diagnostic information. Neither diarrhea nor constipation indicates a neoplasm in the colon. What is significant is a sudden, recent change in bowel habits, frequently a tendency to constipation.

It is a tragic fact that diagnosis of cancer of the rectum and colon is usually made too late to help the patient. If you carefully follow the plan outlined in this book and routinely do rectal, proctosigmoidoscopic, and stool examinations and a barium enema X-ray in all patients with chronic diarrhea or unexplained recent changes in bowel habits, this tragedy could be avoided.

Bibliography

Eisenberg HL, Holb LH, Yam LT, et al: Villous adenoma of the rectum associated with electrolyte disturbance. *Ann Surg* 159:604, 1964

SUMMARY

Benign tumors of the rectum and colon do not usually cause troublesome diarrhea, except for the villous adenoma, which produces large amounts of mucus and has a high tendency to become malignant. It also secretes large amounts of water and electrolytes. At one point in its growth it may cause severe watery diarrhea of 15 to 20 stools in 24 hours. The diagnosis is made by rectal palpation and proctosigmoidoscopic biopsy. The treatment is surgical. Malignant tumors of the right colon cause anemia and a palpable mass; those of the left colon, rectal bleeding and obstruction. Diarrhea is not significant in either. Suspicion must arise if there is a sudden change in bowel habit—most often in the direction of constipation.

Diarrhea from fecal impaction

38

This title sounds contradictory.
Some clinicians prefer the name
pseudodiarrhea. It is not only a real problem but a common
one and is found especially in hospitalized geriatric and psychiatric patients. Pediatricians see it in children with psychogenic megacolon or Hirschsprung's disease.

The symptoms are frequent desire to defecate accompanied by tenesmus, pelvic pain with frequent defecation,
and leaking of liquid feces. Sometimes the condition causes
prolapse of the rectal mucosa and rectal ulcers.

Without a rectal examination, you may conclude that this
is true diarrhea, even dysentery, and prescribe antidiarrheal medication, which of course makes the condition

worse. Frequent examples of this unpardonable error are seen especially in hospital patients who are severely ill, weak, and confined to bed. Fecal impactions occur when medical and nursing personnel are negligent about keeping careful records of patients' intestinal function. Old people develop rectal impaction because they lack good muscle tone in the rectum. Patients with anal lesions may avoid having a bowel movement regularly because of the pain it causes. Psychiatric patients, especially, may retain feces for long periods of time and develop enormous impactions. We have seen this problem in children and adolescents.

Diagnosis is made by rectal palpation. Treatment consists of breaking up the impaction; this often has to be done manually. The mass is broken on rectal examination, followed by an injection via a rubber bulb connected to a catheter of 150-200 ml of warm mineral oil or olive oil as a six-hour or all-night retention enema. This should be followed by an enema of 100 ml of oil and 100 ml of glycerin. Very rarely, the impaction is so hard that it has to be removed surgically.

After the impaction has been removed, measures must be taken to prevent its recurrence and to correct rectal constipation. In old, very weak patients, especially those who are bedridden, there is nothing better than periodic enemas with nonirritating liquids such as mineral oil or normal saline.

Disaccharidase and lactase deficiency

Disaccharidase deficiency

39

From the beginning of the 20th century, a type of flatulent dyspepsia in adults, similar to what was then known as "acid diarrhea in infants," was recognized. The dyspepsia was related to excessive fermentation of carbohydrates in the intestine while other foods, especially proteins, were digested quite normally. Many theories were advanced, but none satisfactorily explained what happened.

The clinical picture, however, is clear and well defined. The patient has chronic diarrhea with two to six stools a day. Considerable borborygmi with minimal or no abdominal pain precede defecation. The expulsion of feces is accompanied by much gas. The gas is usually odorless and is expelled at other times also. The feces are like cereal gruel in consistency and are light yellow. They contain gas bubbles, which make them look foamy, especially if they are inspected some time after they are passed. The odor is sour rather than fetid, something like vinegar. The pH is acid. The patient's general health is not particularly affected, and his appetite continues good. Physical examination is negative except for slight tenderness, slight muscular rigidity, and borborygmi on palpating the abdomen.

Diagnosis could be made by examining the stool after placing the patient on a test diet. Microscopic examination shows much starch and an "iodophilic" flora made up of clostridia and lactobacilli. The decisive study is the "Strasburger fermentation test," which consists of incubating the stools at 38°C for 24 hours. This produces vigorous fermentation, giving off large quantities of gas, and increased acidity of the stool.

Some time ago pediatricians studied acid diarrhea of babies and found that disaccharides were responsible, since eliminating them from the diet resulted in prompt relief. Absorption curves of disaccharides were flat and disaccharides were found undigested in the stool. Monosaccharides resulting from the hydrolysis of the same disaccharides were absorbed normally, as evidenced by their absorption curves.

Two decades ago, our understanding of this problem became clear thanks to two advances: clarification of the mechanism of digestion and absorption of the disaccharides and peroral small intestinal biopsy. In 1961 it was proved that the disaccharidases are found in the brush borders of epithelial cells, where they carry on their digestive action. It was also found that the membrane covering the microvilli takes part in digestion and absorption of food (Chapter 4).

Since peroral biopsy of the small intestine has come into common use, the enzymatic defect is no longer investigated in inert enteric juice containing only desquamated epithelial cells and their enzymes, but more profitably in biopsied mucosa. The defect has been demonstrated directly by measuring the enzymatic action of biopsied epithelial cells in vitro. Basically, the technique consists of incubating the homogenized material with specific substrates and then determining the amount of glucose liberated by means of the glucose oxidase test.

Lactase deficiency

Lactase deficiency in children is characterized by chronic diarrhea with liquid stools containing a high concentration of lactic acid and other organic acids, with a consequent low pH, abnormal lactose tolerance curve, and, sometimes, lactosuria. In adults the clinical picture is more benign: moderate diarrhea, borborygmi, and colicky abdominal pain following the ingestion of milk and its derivatives. The stools are liquid, foamy, and sour smelling with a low pH. At first this deficiency was considered rare, but it's now known to be quite common. Often it is subclinical and there are no symptoms unless the patient oversteps the bounds of his lactose tolerance by taking more milk or milk products than usual. Lactase deficiency varies according to ethnic groups. It is found in only 6 per cent of North American caucasians and is likewise rare in Nordic Europeans. It is common, however, in American and African blacks, American Indians, Asians, and Jews.

Two tests useful in screening for carbohydrate malabsorption should be performed: determination of stool pH and examination for an osmotic gap in the stool fluid. Stool pH is often low in lactase and other disaccharidase deficiencies because of bacterial production of short-chain fatty acids. It is easy to measure with ordinary pH paper. As mentioned in Chapter 2, in osmotic diarrheas the fluid has an osmolarity much higher than twice the sum of sodium and potassium concentrations because other solutes besides these ions (such as short-chain fatty acids) account for a significant fraction of osmolarity.

Four tests are useful in confirming the diagnosis: the lactose tolerance curve, X-ray studies, enzymatic measurements in the mucosa, and, more recently, the breath hydrogen test. The lactose tolerance test was described in Chapter 19. Its diagnostic value has been disputed. Bayless and col-

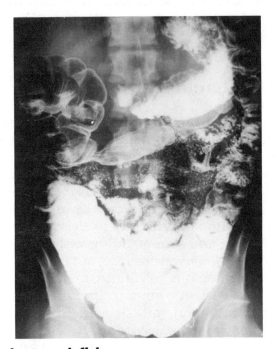

FIGURE 39-1   **Lactase deficiency**
The patient swallowed a mixture of barium and 50 gm of lactose. The radiopaque column reached the cecum in 15 minutes. Bacterial fermentation of the lactose produced gas, which can be seen in the ascending colon

leagues have made the five recommendations that are listed in Chapter 19.

X-rays are very useful and may suffice for diagnosing lactase deficiency without the lactose tolerance test. In lactase deficiency, X-rays of the small intestine look normal following a barium swallow. But if 4 oz of liquid micro-opaque barium sulfate, free from hydrophilic matter, are mixed with 25 gm of lactose, a series of abnormalities appear: dilution of the barium, distention of the loops, and rapid transit of the barium, which reaches the colon in less than an hour (Figure 39-1).

The demonstration of diastase-like action in vitro with tissue from the small intestine is, without doubt, the most direct and precise test, but it is not applicable in general practice. The technique involves incubating homogenized tissue obtained by biopsy with specific substrates, followed by measurement of the glucose liberated by glucose oxidase. Normal subjects have a marked gradient of disaccharidase activity, ranging from low in the duodenum to high in the jejunum and proximal ileum. Patients with lactase deficiency have a low level of this enzyme throughout the intestine.

A means of diagnosing carbohydrate malabsorption that appears to be almost as accurate as direct enzymatic assay is the breath hydrogen test, which depends on colonic fermentation of unabsorbed carbohydrates to hydrogen gas and subsequent absorption and excretion of hydrogen in the lungs. The test is performed by collecting expired air and determining its hydrogen content by gas chromatography before and after the administration of lactose. Because this test is both reliable and noninvasive, it will probably be increasingly used as a test of carbohydrate malabsorption.

Treatment by completely avoiding milk and milk products controls the disease within a few days. This is not easy to do in daily life but, fortunately, reducing the intake and keeping it within the patient's tolerance may be enough. Theoretically, lactase by mouth should be effective. However, lactase is destroyed by gastric juices, and the enzymatic action should take place in the brush border rather than intraluminally. Lactose-free milk may become widely available. It is already in use in some places. Lactase-containing tablets (Lactaid) added to milk hydrolyze the lactose at refrigerator temperatures in 24 hours, converting it to glucose and galactose.

Secondary disaccharidase or lactase deficiencies may follow viral and bacterial gastroenteritis. Omitting disaccharides or lactose from the diet controls the symptoms. Usually the deficiency subsides along with the gastroenteritis, but there are some patients who continue to have intestinal symptoms, especially diarrhea, for days and even weeks unless they avoid the foods they lack the enzymes to digest.

Deficiencies of sucrase and isomaltase are discussed in Chapter 5.

Bibliography

Bayless TM, Rosensweig NS, Christopher N, et al: Milk intolerance and lactose tolerance tests. *Gastroenterology* 54:475, 1968

Bond JH, Levitt MD: Use of breath hydrogen (H_2) in the study of carbohydrate absorption. *Am J Dig Dis* 22:379, 1977

Dahlquist A: The intestinal disaccharidases and disaccharidase intolerance. *Gastroenterology* 43:694, 1962

Dahlquist A, Hammond JB, Crane RK, et al: Intestinal lactase deficiency and lactose intolerance in adults. *Gastroenterology* 45:488, 1963

Gray GM: Intestinal digestion and maldigestion of dietary carbohydrate. *Am Rev Med* 22:391, 1971

Hersh T: Lactose intolerance in health and disease. *Nutr News* Apr 1972, no 2

Laws JW, Spencer J, Neal G: Radiology in the diagnosis of disaccharidase deficiency. *Br J Radiol* 40:594, 1967

Levitt MD, Donaldson RM: Use of respiratory hydrogen (H_2) excretion to detect carbohydrate malabsorption. *J Lab Clin Med* 75:937, 1965

Littman A, Hammond JB: Diarrhea in adults caused by deficiency in intestinal disaccharidase. *Gastroenterology* 48:237, 1965

Weser E, Rubin W, Ross L, et al: Lactase deficiency in patients with the irritable bowel syndrome. *N Engl J Med* 273:1070, 1965

SUMMARY

Disaccharidase deficiency manifests with diarrhea of two to six stools per day, light-colored feces with the consistency of gruel, borborygmi, and much odorless gas on defecation and at other times. The stools contain gas bubbles and have a sour, vinegary odor and an acid pH. The physical examination is essentially negative. The diagnosis is made by stool examination with the patient on a test diet. The microscope shows much starch, clostridia, and lactobacilli. The Strasburger fermentation test results in fermentation with the escape of much gas and an increased acidity of the stool. Since the disaccharidases are found in the brush border of mucosal cells, biopsied mucosa should be measured for enzymatic activity.

Lactase deficiency is quite common in children, manifesting with chronic diarrhea of liquid stools with a low pH and high in lactic acid. Here the lactose tolerance test is abnormal. Four tests confirm the diagnosis: lactose tolerance, X-ray studies, enzymatic measurement of the mucosa, and breath hydrogen. The treatment is avoidance of milk and all its products unless they are free of lactose.

Celiac sprue

40

Celiac sprue is an intestinal disease characterized by malabsorption, typical mucosal lesions, and improvement on avoiding all cereals containing gluten. It is also called idiopathic steatorrhea, nontropical sprue, adult celiac disease, gluten enteropathy, and, in children, celiac disease. Celiac sprue seems to be the most generally used name.

Histopathology

The histopathology of sprue has been known for only about 20 years. The development of the peroral biopsy has permitted a better understanding of the disease. The histologic findings are described in Chapter 23. The most important are changes in the mucosa of the small intestine, especially in the duodenum, next in the jejunum, and least of all in the ileum. The mucosa, when examined with a lens or dissecting microscope, appears flat and devoid of its normal villi. Microscopic examination confirms the findings of a flat surface and villous flattening. The crypts become abnormally long, with increased cellularity and mitosis. The lamina propria shows increased cellularity and is infiltrated with plasma cells and lymphocytes. Electron microscopy shows shortening and fusion of the villi. These changes indicate a marked reduction in absorptive surface in the small intestine. In addition to this, the digestive enzymes located in the cells covering the villi are decreased in activity. It is not difficult to understand, then, why in celiac sprue there is decreased absorption of practically all nutrients, resulting in a malabsorption syndrome.

A gluten-free diet without wheat, rye, barley, and oats is followed by a return to normal in the intestinal epithelial cells. This may be slow and incomplete, particularly in adults. It is accompanied by definite clinical improvement, but treatment with the gluten-free diet must be lifelong. There is no doubt that gluten in these cereals causes celiac sprue; these patients tolerate corn, rice, and sometimes oatmeal. Appendix E lists commercially available foods suitable for a gluten-free diet.

Pathogenesis

Various theories have been proposed to account for the pathogenesis of the gluten-induced damage: (1) the presence of an enzyme deficiency leading to an inability to digest gluten and to production of a substance that damages the mucosa; (2) the presence of surface receptors that permit binding of gluten to the cell surface, with cell death the result; and (3) an abnormal immunologic reaction, since antigluten antibodies are made in the mucosa and cortisone inhibits the lesion in vivo and in vitro. Genetic studies show a familial pattern of the disease and a preponderance of histocompatibility antigens HLA-B8 and HLA-DW3.

Diagnosis

The clinical picture of celiac sprue is described in Chapter 22 with the laboratory tests that establish a diagnosis of malabsorption syndrome. The pertinent X-ray studies are mentioned there and the importance of biopsies is pointed out, since they show changes characteristic of sprue that make a definite diagnosis possible.

The subsidence of symptoms and the improvement in histologic and laboratory findings following a gluten-free diet are so striking that they constitute a therapeutic diagnosis. This is so true that a lack of improvement on the diet is a powerful argument against the diagnosis of celiac sprue.

To establish the diagnosis beyond doubt it is mandatory, at the outset, to obtain a small intestinal biopsy specimen and to document the characteristic lesion. Some authorities insist that two subsequent biopsy specimens are required to confirm the diagnosis: one obtained three months after starting a gluten-free diet, and one obtained after a gluten challenge for at least two weeks. Since the small intestinal mucosa in children may become flat in a variety of other diseases (such as acute gastroenteritis, cow's milk and soy protein allergy, eosinophilic gastroenteritis, chronic diarrhea of infancy, immunodeficiency disorders, bacterial overgrowth, tropical sprue, and giardiasis), failure to confirm the diagnosis in this manner will result in improper diagnosis in as many as one-third of patients. Such patients are improperly condemned to lifelong gluten restriction.

Treatment

During treatment, make sure the patient is on a strict gluten-free diet. Even very small amounts of gluten cause continued symptoms and relapses. The patient *must* understand this. It is necessary to explain to him that many processed foods can contain wheat: ice cream, salad dressings, canned goods, instant coffee, catsup, mustard, and many candies. Likewise rye, barley, and usually oats must be omitted. Rice flour, cornstarch and corn meal, and soya are tolerated.

Patients with celiac sprue very frequently have also lactose intolerance because of a deficiency in lactase secondary to the enteropathy. On a gluten-free diet the intestinal epithelium tends to return to normal, and with this improvement, the lactase deficiency also improves.

The diet should be supplemented with the necessary amounts of iron, folic acid, vitamin B_{12}, and vitamin K. Dehydrated patients should receive liquids and electrolytes intravenously. The rare cases of tetany are caused by hypocalcemia and/or hypomagnesemia. These patients should be treated with 1 to 2 gm of calcium gluconate and/or 0.5 to 1 gm of magnesium sulfate intravenously. In all cases of hypocalcemia and osteomalacia, calcium lactate or gluconate, 6 gm, and vitamin D, 50,000 units/day, should be given by mouth. Vitamins A, C, E, and B complex should be given also.

Complications

"Refractory sprue" begins as ordinary gluten-sensitive enteropathy, but after some time symptoms and histologic lesions recur despite strict adherence to a gluten-free diet. Fortunately, this condition may respond favorably to corticosteroid therapy. Other complications of celiac sprue are "ulcerative jejunoileitis" and certain malignancies of the gastrointestinal tract, including carcinoma and lymphoma.

Bibliography

Ament ME: Malabsorption syndromes in infancy and childhood. *J Pediatr* 81:585, 867, 1972

Bayless TM, Kaplowitz RF, Shelley WM, et al: Intestinal ulceration as a complication of celiac disease. *N Engl J Med* 236:996, 1967

Falchuk ZM: Update on gluten-sensitive enteropathy. *Am J Med* 67:1085, 1979

Harris OD, Cooke WT, Thompson H, et al: Malignancy in adult celiac disease and idiopathic steatorrhea. *Am J Med* 42:899, 1967

Mann JG, Brown WR, Kern F: The subtle and variable clinical expressions of gluten induced enteropathy. *Am J Med* 48:357, 1970

Pena AS, Mann DL, Hague NE, et al: Genetic basis of gluten sensitive enteropathy. *Gastroenterology* 75:230, 1978

Stokes PL, Asquith P, Holmes GKT, et al: Histocompatibility antigens associated with adult celiac disease. *Lancet* 2:162, 1972

Trier JS, Falchuk ZM, Carey MC, et al: Celiac sprue and refractory sprue. *Gastroenterology* 75:307, 1978

SUMMARY

Celiac sprue (also known as idiopathic steatorrhea, nontropical sprue, adult celiac disease, gluten enteropathy, and, in children, celiac disease) is characterized by intestinal malabsorption and mucosal lesions. It is successfully treated by total gluten avoidance. The typical mucosal changes are flattening of its surface (due to villous shortening and fusion), increased length of crypts, increased cellularity of both crypts and lamina propria, resulting in diminished absorptive surface, and a decrease in absorption of all nutrients. Why gluten produces such damage is unknown. A strict gluten-free diet is not only proper therapy but also a positive diagnostic test where the symptoms disappear. Many other conditions may produce mucosal flattening of the small intestine, especially in children. The gluten-free diet must be strict and supplemented with iron, folic acid, and vitamins B_{12} and K. Other accompanying symptoms must be treated symptomatically. Complications may be "refractory sprue" that responds to corticosteroids, ulcerative jejunoileitis, and various gastrointestinal malignancies.

Tropical sprue

41

Tropical sprue is found frequently in certain parts of the world. It causes a serious malabsorption syndrome and is difficult to diagnose. Its symptoms may be vague and its etiology and pathogenesis are not understood.

Tropical sprue is a syndrome characterized by malabsorption, malnutrition, and structural changes in the mucosa of the small intestine. It may be diagnosed in individuals who live or have lived in endemic areas and who have had other causes of malabsorption ruled out and who respond to prolonged treatment with antibiotics. The disease's etiology is unknown. When it is understood, a better name may be found.

The disease is generally chronic. To call it "tropical" is misleading, since it can occur in the Himalayas and other cold areas. There are also many tropical areas where it does not occur although they may border on regions where it is endemic. It is common in India, Southeast Asia, and in some islands of the West Indies, but not in Jamaica. In the endemic areas there may be neighborhoods and even homes where it is found next door to families who are free of the disease.

The symptoms are diarrhea and steatorrhea with frequent, soft, pasty, voluminous, very fetid stools that are pale, greasy, and frothy. Bowel movements occur both day and night. The patient's abdomen is distended with gas. Borborygmi, abdominal colicky pain, and flatulence are common complaints.

Thanks to laboratory studies it can be proved that all nutrients are poorly absorbed: fats, carbohydrates, proteins, folic acid, vitamins, water, and minerals. Nutritional effects are loss of weight, weakness, pallor, paresthesias, cheilosis, stomatitis, glossitis, hemorrhages, tetany, and subacute combined sclerosis of the spinal cord.

The most important laboratory findings are macrocytic anemia, leukopenia, thrombocytopenia, and megaloblastic bone marrow from vitamin B_{12} and folic acid deficiency; low serum levels of albumin, calcium, magnesium, potassium, phosphates, and carotene; moderately high fecal excretion of fats; a flat D-xylose absorption curve with simultaneous decreased five-hour urinary excretion of this sugar; deficient absorption of B_{12} not corrected by addition of intrinsic factor; and deficient absorption of folates.

X-rays of the small intestine may be normal or may show nonspecific changes found in other malabsorption syndromes (Chapter 20).

Biopsies of the small intestine don't show specific changes either (Chapter 23), but they are useful because they show shortening and thickening of the villi, which tend to fuse and branch. Under the dissecting microscope the mucosa has a foliaceous appearance. The light microscope shows inflammatory infiltration of the mucosa. These changes are seen in many "normal" individuals who live in endemic zones. It's said that the part of a population that is ill with tropical sprue is only the tip of the iceberg formed by those who live under ecologic conditions of bacterial contamination and inadequate food intake.

The onset of tropical sprue may be gradual or sudden. If it is sudden, it's usually blamed on eating spoiled food, acute indigestion, a change of diet, or a trip to some other region. When the tourist or foreigner takes up residence in an endemic area, the initial picture may look like tourist diarrhea. Only its chronicity and the appearance of malnutrition point to the diagnosis.

Clinically, three phases of the disease have been described. In the initial phase the patient complains of bulky stools and fatigue. The second phase occurs after weeks or months with symptoms and signs of malnutrition: weight loss, glossitis, stomatitis, cheilosis, and hypoalbuminemia. The third stage is characterized by severe malnutrition and megaloblastic anemia.

The cause or causes of the disease are unknown. Folate deficiency is probably not the cause but the result of deficient intestinal absorption. There is no intolerance to gluten or to any polypeptide, and a gluten-free diet gives only partial improvement. Many patients have lactose intolerance, but this is concomitant or secondary. One theory is that the disease is caused by excessive proliferation of bacteria in the intestine because the onset often follows an attack of infectious gastroenteritis and because sometimes it occurs in epidemics. Supporters of this theory cite the compatible histologic changes in the intestine. The fact that large numbers of coliform bacteria are found high up in the small intestine and that the patient improves on antibiotics are two strong arguments in support of the theory of bacterial overgrowth. There are, however, arguments against it: Bacteria are not always found in the small intestine, nor do they occur in great numbers; and the improvement with antibiotics is very slow. Many attempts have been made to find an infectious agent: virus, *Mycoplasma* bacteria, fungi, algae, protozoa. Recently *Klebsiella oxytoca (pneumoniae)* and *Enterobacter cloacae* have been suspected. *E. cloacae* and serotypes 1, 2, and 5 of *K. oxytoca* produce toxins that cause secretory diarrhea and changes in the epithelium that resemble those seen in tropical sprue. The theory is attractive but does not satisfy Koch's postulates.

Treatment is the administration of broad-spectrum antibiotics. Tetracycline is preferred, but nonabsorbable sulfonamides have been found effective. Tetracycline, 250 mg four times a day for six months or longer, gradually restores clinical, biochemical, and histologic findings to normal, especially if the patient leaves the endemic zone and avoids relapses or reinfection. If that is not possible—and usually it is not—the abnormal laboratory and histologic findings persist or return.

Folic acid and vitamin B_{12} are extremely effective in correcting the anemia and, in many patients, also relieve the intestinal symptoms and improve absorptive function and mucosal morphology.

Bibliography

Baker SJ, Mathan VI, Joseph I: Epidemic tropical sprue. *Am J Dig Dis* 7:959, 1962

Gorbach SL, Mitra R, Jacobs B, et al: Bacterial contamination of the upper small bowel in tropical sprue. *Lancet* 1:74, 1969

Klipstein FA: Tropical sprue. *Gastroenterology* 54:275, 1968

Klipstein FA, Engert RF, Short HB: Enterotoxigenicity of colonising coliform bacteria in tropical sprue and blind-loop syndrome. *Lancet* 2:342, 1978

Klipstein FA, Holdeman LV, Corcino JJ, et al: Enterotoxigenic intestinal bacteria in tropical sprue. *Ann Intern Med* 79:632, 1973

Lindenbaum J: Tropical enteropathy. *Gastroenterology* 64:637, 1973

Lindenbaum J: Aspects of vitamin B_{12} and folate metabolism in malabsorption syndromes. *Am J Med* 67:1037, 1979

Swanson VL, Thomassen RW: Pathology of the jejunal mucosa in tropical sprue. *Am J Pathol* 46:511, 1965

Tomkins AM, James WPT, Drasar BS: Bacterial colonisation of jejunal mucosa in acute tropical sprue. *Lancet* 1:59, 1975

SUMMARY

Tropical sprue is a chronic malabsorption syndrome that is common in India, Southeast Asia, the West Indies (not in Jamaica), and other areas, not necessarily tropical. The symptoms are diarrhea, steatorrhea, frequent, fetid, pasty, frothy stools occurring day and night, distended abdomen, borborygmi, colicky pain, and flatulence. The onset is sudden or gradual and occurs in three phases. The first phase is bulky stools and fatigue. The second, after weeks or months, is malnutrition, weight loss, glossitis, stomatitis, cheilosis, and hypoglobulinemia. The third is severe malnutrition and megaloblastic anemia. All nutrients are poorly absorbed. The cause of this condition is unknown although it is suspected that proliferation of bacteria in the intestine may be responsible. The treatment is tetracycline or nonabsorbable sulfonamides, folic acid, and vitamin B_{12}.

Intestinal tuberculosis

42

Before streptomycin revolution-
ized the treatment and prognosis
of tuberculosis, the judgment of Hippocrates was correct:
"Patients with tuberculosis . . . who develop diarrhea will
die. Diarrhea in patients with tuberculosis is a mortal symptom." Fortunately, thanks to antibiotics and chemotherapy,
intestinal tuberculosis is rare now and does not carry the
grave prognosis of former years.

Intestinal tuberculosis has been divided morphologically
into three varieties: ulcerative, hypertrophic, and ulcerohypertrophic. Ulcerative tuberculosis is nearly always secondary to pulmonary tuberculosis and is produced by swallowed bacteria. The hypertrophic and ulcerohypertrophic

varieties are much less common than ulcerative tuberculosis. They occur without pulmonary tuberculosis and are attributed to primary infection with the bovine strain of the tubercle bacillus.

Secondary intestinal tuberculosis

Secondary intestinal tuberculosis is a chronic enterocolitis produced by the invasion of bacilli from open pulmonary lesions or, less frequently, from extension of tuberculous lesions in the female internal genitalia. The capsule of the bacillus protects it from the action of gastric juice and it reaches the intestine, where it preferentially attacks the ileocecal region but may lodge anywhere. Achlorhydria favors infection of the intestine with tuberculosis. The initial inflammatory reaction takes place in the lymph follicles and Peyer's patches and is followed by sloughing of the mucosa and formation of ulcers with irregular undermined borders. The fibrotic reaction produces adhesions to adjoining loops and intestinal retraction with narrowing of the lumen. Edema, cellular infiltration, and lymphatic hyperplasia all contribute to thickening of the intestinal walls. Tubercles form, grow, and eventually reach the serosa. The bacilli travel through the lymphatics to the mesenteric lymph nodes, where they produce hyperplasia, caseous necrosis, and calcification. In the late stages the lymphatics are obstructed and inflammatory masses, made up of intestinal loops, thickened mesentery, and adhesions, form. Microscopic examination reveals infiltration by mononuclear cells, epithelioid reaction, and the characteristic caseous necrosis that differentiates tuberculosis from regional enteritis and other granulomatous processes of the intestine. Caseous necrosis may be limited to the mesenteric lymph nodes. Finding these and, better still, identifying the tubercle bacillus by means of special staining methods and cultures are essential to the diagnosis.

The clinical picture of secondary tuberculosis of the intestine consists of diarrhea, abdominal pain, anorexia, and weight loss. The diarrhea is typical of inflammatory and ulcerative enteropathies and consists of four to six soft or semiliquid stools a day with mucus, but rarely with pus or blood. If the process involves much of the intestine, if there is lymphatic obstruction, or if the absorption of bile salts is greatly impaired, steatorrhea and other symptoms of malabsorption result. The abdominal pain is caused by narrowing and partial occlusion of the intestinal lumen and is felt in the periumbilical area or in the right lower quadrant. The pain is colicky and is relieved by vomiting or defecation. It generally occurs immediately after eating, which makes the patient afraid to eat. This, combined with anorexia, contributes to rapid weight loss and debility.

In addition to general poor health and the signs of pulmonary tuberculosis, physical examination reveals tenderness in the right lower abdominal quadrant, sometimes with muscular guarding, and, in about half the cases, a palpable painful mass in the ileocecal region.

Rectal and sigmoidoscopic examinations are usually negative, except in cases of rectosigmoid tuberculosis, where there are large transverse ulcers with irregular undermined borders. X-ray findings are described in detail in Chapter 20. They may be very helpful but, even so, a differential diagnosis excluding regional enteritis, lymphoma, actinomycosis, and even amebiasis of the cecum may be very difficult.

The intradermal tuberculin test is not of much value here. A positive reaction does not make the diagnosis, and a negative reaction does not rule it out, though it makes tuberculosis less likely. The only way to make a definite diagnosis is to find caseous necrosis in the intestinal walls or mesenteric lymph nodes or, even better, to find acid-fast tubercle bacilli in stained preparations of tissue or in cultures, or to obtain positive findings following animal inoculation with material taken during surgery.

Primary intestinal tuberculosis

Primary intestinal tuberculosis is rarely diagnosed nowadays. This is not only because the disease is becoming very rare but also because regional enteritis is less frequently misdiagnosed as tuberculosis. We cannot, however, disregard primary intestinal tuberculosis completely, since it does exist. It is usually found in the ileocecal area but, like secondary tuberculosis, can occur in any part of the intestine. When it affects the terminal ileum and the cecum, the walls become very thick, the lumen narrows, and the mucosa hypertrophies and becomes ulcerated. Microscopically, extensive round-cell infiltration and marked hyperplasia of fibrous tissue are seen. There are multiple granulomas, characterized by epithelioid cells, giant cells, and central caseous necrosis of the tubercles.

Primary intestinal tuberculosis is difficult to distinguish from regional enteritis, ameboma, sarcoid, mycosis, nonspecific granulomas, and cancer. Often histologic examination of tissue following surgical removal will give the diagnosis. Diarrhea is less common in this type of intestinal tuberculosis than in the secondary, or ulcerative, type. Obstructive symptoms are more common. A negative hemagglutination reaction for amebiasis rules out ameboma. Simultaneous involvement of the cecum and terminal ileum makes cancer improbable. X-ray findings are discussed in Chapter 20. Colonoscopy is probably valuable, but experience with it in patients with intestinal tuberculosis is lacking.

Treatment

The best treatment of tuberculosis is begun with three primary drugs: streptomycin, isoniazid (INH), and ethambutol (Myambutol). Streptomycin is withdrawn after three to six months. Isoniazid and ethambutol are continued for at least a year, followed by another year with isoniazid alone.

It's sometimes necessary to resort to surgery for diagnostic purposes or to relieve obstruction. When the histologic examination has established the diagnosis, surgical treatment should be supplemented by the chemotherapy and antibiotic treatment outlined above. The diarrhea and malnutrition should of course be treated with adequate diet, omitting fats and substituting medium-chain triglycerides in cases of steatorrhea and adding parenteral supplements. Some patients with intestinal tuberculosis lose proteins from the intestine and therefore need protein supplements.

Bibliography

American JL, Martin JD: Tuberculosis of the alimentary tract. *Am J Surg* 107:340, 1964

Bentley G, Webster JHH: Gastrointestinal tuberculosis. *Br J Surg* 54:90, 1967

Bondurant RE, Reid D: Ileocecal tuberculosis. *Am J Gastroenterol* 63:58, 1975

Chuttani HK: Intestinal tuberculosis. *Mod Trends Gastroenterol* 309, 1970

Schulze K, Warner HA, Murray D: Intestinal tuberculosis. Experience at a Canadian teaching institution. *Am J Med* 63:735, 1977

SUMMARY

One variety of intestinal tuberculosis is ulcerative, occurring secondary to pulmonary tuberculosis via swallowed organisms or occasionally from extension from the female internal genitalia. It manifests clinically with diarrhea, abdominal pain, anorexia, and weight loss. Physical examination reveals poor health, signs of pulmonary tuberculosis, tenderness in the right lower quadrant with or without muscle guarding and with or without a palpable, painful mass in the ileocecal region. It must be differentiated from regional enteritis, lymphoma, actinomycosis, and cecal amebiasis. A positive diagnosis is made on finding the organism in stained preparations of tissue or in material taken from animal inoculation.

Primary tuberculosis, manifesting as the hypertrophic or ulcerohypertrophic variety, is usually found in the ileocecal region but can occur in any part of the intestine. It must be differentiated from amebiasis, sarcoid, mycosis, nonspecific granuloma, and carcinoma. Diarrhea is not too common here, but obstructive symptoms are. The diagnosis often requires surgery, as does the obstruction. The treatment consists of streptomycin, isoniazid (INH), and ethambutol (Myambutol) plus attention to diarrhea and malnutrition.

Regional enteritis

43

Regional enteritis, or Crohn's disease, is a chronic inflammatory disease characterized by edema, thickening of all layers of the intestinal wall, and consequent narrowing of the lumen. The mucosal surface looks cobblestoned because of the many linear ulcers, which may be transverse or longitudinal. Polypoid and ulcerated areas alternate with mucosa of normal appearance. Another characteristic of Crohn's disease is the presence of fistulae that connect the intestinal loops and open into the bladder or other abdominal or pelvic organs or into the abdominal wall. The mesentery is thickened. A striking finding on opening the abdomen is mesenteric fat surrounding the free border of the diseased intestinal segments. The involvement of the mesentery and peritoneal serosa explains the tendency of the loops to adhere and mat together. The mesenteric lymph nodes are inflamed and enlarged.

Microscopically all the layers of the intestinal wall are seen to be inflamed. Granulomas are frequent. These are accumulations of epithelioid cells surrounded by lymphocytes and other mononuclear cells at times including Langhans cells. Unlike tuberculous granulomas, there is no caseation. Other frequent findings are lymphoid hyperplasia, lymphangiectasia, and perilymphangitis as well as deep ulcers separated by areas of normal mucosa.

Crohn's disease may affect any part of the intestine, but it occurs most frequently in the terminal ileum. The sites of involvement vary in size from a few centimeters to several decimeters.

Clinical course

The onset of Crohn's disease is usually in early adult life. It becomes chronic and generally progressive with exacerbations and remissions. The principal symptoms are pain, diarrhea, abdominal mass, bleeding, fistulae and perianal abscesses, fever, weight loss or retarded growth, and anemia. The pain is mesogastric or hypogastric or localized in the right iliac fossa. It's often colicky and relieved by defecation and is due to the narrowing of the intestine. When the pain is constant and not colicky, it's due to the inflammatory mass surrounding the ileum. The diarrhea consists of four to six bowel movements a day, which are not urgent as they are in inflammatory processes in the colon and rectum. The patient has no trouble controlling the moment of defecation. The stools are sometimes liquid but more frequently pasty and rarely bloody. Intestinal hemorrhage of variable size, however, is not rare. In advanced cases a painful mass is usually found in the right iliac fossa and consists of thickened, matted loops of the intestine.

Sometimes the first symptom of the disease is pseudoappendicular pain. At other times it is an anal fistula that is resistant to treatment, or a chronic indurated anal fissure. Fistulae may open into the abdominal wall, into loops of the small or large intestine, and into the bladder or the vagina. Fever, anemia, weight loss, and, in children and adolescents, retarded growth are other important manifestations of this serious illness.

The course of Crohn's disease varies greatly from one individual to another. Some patients suffer a few episodes of diarrhea and have no further trouble the rest of their lives. In others the disease is progressive, continuous, and beset with complications. The most common course is chronic and prolonged with exacerbations and remissions, and the eventual development of complications that require surgery. The most common complications are acute and chronic intestinal obstruction, fistulae, hemorrhage, migratory polyarthritis, iritis, erythema nodosum, deformity of the fingers (clubbed fingers), amyloidosis, and a tendency to develop gallstones and urinary calculi. Malnutrition and cachexia are common as a result of anorexia, fear of eating because of the pain it causes, ill-advised dietary restrictions, deficient intestinal absorption, and impaired absorption of bile salts and vitamin B_{12}, which ordinarily takes place in the terminal part of the ileum.

Diagnosis

The disease is most common among Jews and persons of Northern European extraction. It should be considered as a diagnostic possibility in all young adults who complain of persistent diarrhea, especially if accompanied by abdominal pain and slight fever. X-ray studies are the most important diagnostic procedures, described in Chapter 20. Differential diagnosis includes lymphoma and intestinal tuberculosis. Tuberculosis may be difficult to rule out, especially in the absence of pulmonary symptoms. Then histopathologic studies of the involved tissue—necessitating surgery—are needed to make the diagnosis.

The cause of Crohn's disease is not known. No infectious agent has been identified. The special way the host reacts to the pathogenic agent in inflammatory and immunologic responses may be of great importance. An inherited constitutional predisposition is suspected. The role of emotional factors in pathogenesis remains undefined.

Treatment

Unfortunately, there is no effective treatment for Crohn's disease. Therapy is limited to preventing or correcting the malnutrition by means of a well-balanced diet, avoiding irritating and high-residue foods, giving elemental diets where there is deficient intestinal absorption (see Chapter 44), supplementing the diet with parenteral solutions, symptomatic treatment with antispasmodics and antidiarrheals, and decreasing the inflammation with adrenal steroids.

Steroids should be given only if all other measures fail because of their side effects and other dangers and because they are not curative. Prednisone in moderately high doses (80 mg/day in adults) is commonly used. The dose is gradually reduced, depending on the therapeutic response, until it is discontinued where possible. Many clinicians prefer ACTH intravenously, maintaining that they get better results with it. It is possible that prednisone is not well absorbed by the inflamed mucosa of the intestine. In any case, when the patient receives adequate doses of either ACTH or prednisone, the diarrhea usually rapidly improves and the fever and other symptoms subside.

Unfortunately, it is not possible to prevent the relapses or the complications. Steroids do not cure the disease. Sulfasalazine has been used, but its therapeutic value is doubtful. A recent controlled trial suggests that sulfasalazine and prednisone are both more effective than placebos in diminishing the clinical features of active Crohn's disease.

Immunosuppressive drugs (azathioprine, 6-mercaptopurine) have been tried, with promising results in some cases.

Surgical treatment is reserved for complications: intestinal obstruction that does not respond to intubation and steroids, recurring hemorrhage, external fistulae, and retarded development. Surgery is also indicated when all conservative methods have failed and the patient is becoming a chronic invalid. Reluctance to recommend surgical proce-dures is due to the fact that all of them—short circuits, sim-ple anastomoses, or resection of the affected segments—are eventually followed by relapses. It's impossible to predict how soon they will occur. Eventually, many patients with regional enteritis suffer a dangerous reduction in the ab-sorptive capacity of their intestine because of extensive dam-age to the mucosa or because of surgery. The serious nutri-tional problems that arise under these circumstances have been partly solved by two outstanding advances: parenteral alimentation (Appendix F) and elemental diets (Chapter 44).

Bibliography

Donaldson RM: Crohn's disease of the small bowel. In *Gastrointestinal Disease* (Sleisenger MH, Fordtran JS, eds), 2nd ed, p 1052. Philadelphia: Saunders, 1978

Farmer RG, Hawk WA, Turnbull RB: Clinical patterns in Crohn's disease: A statistical study of 615 patients. *Gastroenterology* 68:627, 1975

Greenstein AJ, Sacher DB, Pasternak BS, et al: Reoperation and recur-rence in Crohn's colitis and ileocolitis. *N Engl J Med* 293:685, 1975

Koltz U, Maier K, Fischer C, et al: Therapeutic efficacy of sulfasalazine and its metabolites in patients with ulcerative colitis and Crohn's dis-ease. *N Engl J Med* 303:1499, 1980

Present DH, Korelitz BI, Wisch N, et al: Treatment of Crohn's disease with 6-mercaptopurine. *N Engl J Med* 302:981, 1980

Singleton JW: National Cooperative Crohn's Disease Study. Results of drug treatment (abstr). *Gastroenterology* 72:1133, 1977

SUMMARY

Regional enteritis, or Crohn's disease, is chronic and in-flammatory with edema, thickening of all layers of the intes-tinal wall, narrowing of its lumen, and many linear ulcers that give the mucosa a cobblestone appearance. Polypoid areas and ulcers alternate with normal mucosa. Fistulae connect intestinal loops, open into the abdominal wall or pel-vic or abdominal organs, and involve the mesentery and peritoneal serosa. The mesenteric lymph nodes are inflamed, and noncaseating granulomas are not uncommon. Although any part of the intestine may be involved, the most common area is the terminal ileum.

The cause is unknown. The condition usually comes on in early adult life and is progressive with remissions and eventual chronicity. It manifests with pain, diarrhea, bleeding, fever, weight loss or retarded growth, abdominal mass, fistulae, and perianal abscesses. The most common complications are intestinal obstruction, hemorrhage, migratory polyarthritis, iritis, erythema nodosum, clubbed fingers, amyloidosis, gall- and kidney stones, malnutrition, and cachexia. The differential diagnosis includes lymphomas and intestinal tuberculosis. The treatment is entirely nonspecific (steroids), with surgery for the complications.

Short bowel syndrome

44

Marked reduction of the functional area of the small intestine gives rise to clinical and laboratory findings that are called the short bowel syndrome. It is the result of surgical resections or short circuits, which are being done more often and more skillfully because of advances in surgery.

Resections and short circuits are done in mesenteric thrombosis, abdominal trauma, regional enteritis, intestinal obstruction with strangulation, intestinal cancer, radiation enteropathy, and malignant obesity (jejunoileal bypass). The survival and quality of life of the patient depend on the ability of the remaining intestine to digest and absorb and on the quality of medical care.

The functional capacity of the intestine depends on the length of the part remaining, its location, its functional integrity and capacity to adapt, presence or absence of the ileocecal valve, and the functional integrity of the other digestive organs.

The remaining intestine

The length of the part not removed or bypassed is of great importance. Survival is unusual if less than 60 cm are left. Nutritional problems are in inverse proportion to the amount of intestine remaining. The ileum may take over the work of the jejunum by absorbing carbohydrates, proteins, and fats, but both the ileum and the jejunum have specialized functions. The jejunum absorbs iron and calcium most efficiently, and the ileum selectively absorbs bile salts and vitamin B_{12}. Failure to absorb bile salts produces biliary insufficiency, resulting in malabsorption of lipids and diarrhea. Deficient absorption of B_{12} gives rise to megaloblastic anemia.

Functional integrity

The functional integrity of the remaining intestine is of great importance in the postoperative prognosis. For example, if the rest of the small intestine and the colon are normal, the problem is less difficult than if the small intestine is diseased, as in regional enteritis, or if part or all of the colon has been removed. Likewise, the functional state of the liver and pancreas are important in prognosis.

Capacity to adapt

The regenerative powers of the intestine play an important role. Although the nonfunctioning part atrophies, the functioning part experiences hyperplasia and its absorptive powers gradually increase. Nutrients in the lumen of the small intestine are required to stimulate the process of intestinal adaptation. This stimulation may be mediated via direct mucosal absorption or metabolism of nutrients, by the presence of pancreatobiliary secretions in the intestine, by trophic effects of circulating enteric hormones, or by neurovascular influences.

Ileocecal valve

When the ileocecal valve has to be removed surgically, diarrhea becomes more severe. The valve blocks the ascent of bacteria from the colon to the small intestine. Without this valve, bacteria reach the ileum in great numbers and cause the bacterial overgrowth syndrome. Bacteria colonizing the small intestine are considered responsible for consuming vitamin B_{12} and changing the chemical structure of the bile salts by deconjugating and dehydroxylating them. This causes steatorrhea.

Complications

Following intestinal resection, gastric secretion increases considerably for some time because the normal inactivation of gastrin by the small bowel is partly lost. This increased activity may cause peptic ulcer, diarrhea from increased secretion, and inactivation of pancreatic enzymes with consequent steatorrhea.

Another possible complication is the formation of calcium oxalate kidney stones as a result of excessive absorption of oxalates from food. Normally, oxalates combine with calcium to form insoluble salts, but when there is steatorrhea the calcium combines with fatty acids, forming soaps, and the oxalic acid is absorbed.

Management

Management of the patient with short intestine during the first stage, lasting two or three weeks, includes parenteral feedings with adequate intake of calories, electrolytes, and water. Diarrhea is controlled with codeine, paregoric, or diphenoxylate. Effects of gastric hypersecretion can be controlled with anticholinergics, antacids, and, particularly, the new potent antihistamine H_2 blocker cimetidine

(Tagamet). Feeding by mouth should be started slowly and carefully, taking several months to discontinue parenteral feedings completely.

Fortunately, elemental diets are available. They contain well-balanced mixtures of amino acids, carbohydrates, and sometimes medium-chain triglycerides, making absorption easy for the remaining intestine. Their unpleasant taste may make it necessary to give them by nasogastric catheter. They should be given in dilute solutions because otherwise their hyperosmolarity would cause diarrhea. The final aim is, of course, to get the patient back on oral feedings. Frequent small meals containing very little fat are recommended. They should be supplemented by calcium and magnesium salts, fat-soluble vitamins A, D, and K, vitamin B_{12}, and often folic acid and the water-soluble vitamins. Lactase deficiency is common, so it's wise to omit milk and milk products.

In cases of resection limited to the terminal ileum, vitamin B_{12} should be given parenterally. Diarrhea may occur from the action of unabsorbed bile salts on the mucosa of the colon. The resin cholestyramine sequesters bile salts and may prove very effective given in doses of 12 to 16 gm/day. If the intestinal resection has been extensive and there is steatorrhea, cholestyramine is contraindicated because reducing the available bile salts makes the steatorrhea worse.

Patients who have had the ileocecal valve removed and develop an overgrowth of bacteria in the remaining intestine, with resulting diarrhea, can be treated with broad-spectrum antibiotics such as tetracycline and ampicillin. Unfortunately, the relief is only temporary.

Surgical variations

New surgical procedures have been attempted, such as interposing antiperistaltic loops and constructing anastomoses that allow the intestinal contents to travel in circles through the same loops in order to prolong contact with the intestinal wall and so aid absorption. Results have not been good.

Recently, what has been called euphemistically an artificial intestine has come into use. By means of an implanted arteriovenous fistula or a Silastic atrial catheter, the patient receives intravenously, for 12 hours every night, a solution of nutrients designed to allow normal nutrition to be maintained during the months required for bowel adaptation to occur. Because bowel adaptation to the absorption and transport of foodstuffs depends in part on the intraluminal presence of foodstuffs, elemental and regular diets are ingested during the period of intravenous support, which may last for years. By using combined oral and intravenous nutrition, approximately 20 per cent of patients with short bowel syndrome eventually can take sufficient oral nutrients to sustain life.

Bibliography

Buxton B: Small bowel resection and gastric hypersecretion. *Gut* 15:229, 1974

Compston JE, Creamer B: The consequences of small intestinal resection. *Q J Med* 46:485, 1977

Cortot A, Flemming CR, Malagelada JR: Improved nutrient absorption after cimetidine in short bowel syndrome with gastric hypersecretion. *N Engl J Med* 300:79, 1979

Dobbins JW, Binder HJ: Importance of the colon in enteric hyperoxaluria. *N Engl J Med* 296:298, 1977

Levine JM, Deren JJ, Yezdimir E: Small bowel resection. Oral intake is the stimulus for hyperplasia. *Dig Dis* 21:542, 1976

Scribner BH, Riella MC: The "artificial gut system" for home parenteral nutrition. *Gastroenterology* 68:983, 1975

Sheldon GF: Role of parenteral nutrition in patients with short bowel syndrome. *Am J Med* 67:1021, 1979

Strauss E, Gerson CD, Yallow RS: Hypersecretion of gastrin associated with the short bowel syndrome. *Gastroenterology* 66:175, 1974

Weser E: The management of patients after small bowel resection. *Gastroenterology* 71:146, 1976

Weser E: Nutritional aspects of malabsorption. Short gut adaptation. *Am J Med* 67:1014, 1979

Williamson RCN: Medical progress: Intestinal adaptation. Structural, functional and cytokinetic changes. *N Engl J Med* 298:1393, 1444, 1978

SUMMARY

Short bowel syndrome is due to reduction of the functional area of the small intestine by surgical resection or short circuits. The functional capacity of the remaining gut depends on its length and location. Survival is unusual if less than 60 cm remain. The functioning part of the remnant small intestine undergoes hyperplasia and gradually increases its absorptive power. Management during the first two to three postoperative weeks includes parenteral feeding with adequate calories, water, and electrolytes and treatment with antidiarrheals, anticholinergics, antacids, and cimetidine (Tagamet) to control gastric hypersecretion. Oral feeding is introduced slowly over several months, with frequent small meals containing little fat, calcium and magnesium salts, vitamins A, D, K, and B_{12}, folic acid, and the water-soluble vitamins. With combined oral and IV nutrition, 20 per cent of patients eventually can take sufficient oral nutrients to sustain life.

Whipple's disease

45

Whipple's disease, or intestinal lipodystrophy, is so rare that most gastroenterologists see only a few cases in their entire careers. It was described by Whipple in 1907 as follows: "Up until now this disease has not been recognized. Anatomically it is characterized by deposits of fat and fatty acids in the lymphatic tissue of the intestine and the mesentery." Whipple described extensive infiltration of the lamina propria with macrophages, the spongy appearance of the cytoplasm of these cells, the large lipoid deposits in the lamina propria and mesenteric lymph nodes, and changes in the structure of the villi. He also found small, rod-shaped organisms less than 2 μm long in the lamina propria. Only the following has been added to his description: (1) Similar histologic lesions have also been found in many other organs and tissues, including peripheral lymph nodes, liver, spleen, heart valves, lungs, kidneys, adrenal glands, bone, and central nervous system; (2) the macrophages contain many glucoprotein granules that can be stained with periodic acid-Schiff (PAS); and (3) the small, rod-shaped organisms are bacilli. The etiologic significance of the bacilli in this disease is not understood. They do, however, diminish in number as clinical improvement takes place with antibiotics. Their identity and relationship to the pathogenesis are still unknown.

The classical clinical picture of Whipple's disease is made up of a combination of various syndromes: malabsorption, fever, arthritis, and neurologic involvement. The malabsorption syndrome described in Chapter 22 is the same in this disease. Fever occurs in half the cases and is chronic and intermittent. The polyarthritis is inflammatory and migratory, with remission and without sequelae. It attacks the large and medium-sized joints. The neurologic changes are altered memory, orientation, and conduct, and symptoms of both peripheral and central neuropathy: ophthalmoplegia, nystagmus, and facial hypoesthesia. Patients develop diffuse cutaneous pigmentation and generalized enlargement of lymph nodes.

The diagnosis should not be difficult when this combination of syndromes occurs. Unfortunately, they do not appear simultaneously, but one by one over a period of months and even years. The result is that they are diagnosed as fevers of unknown origin, unclassified chronic arthritis, or other poorly understood illnesses.

Laboratory tests show only the nonspecific changes of malabsorption, which do not make a specific diagnosis. X-ray studies of the small intestine may be very helpful. They show marked thickening of the transverse folds of the upper part of the jejunum. Similar thickening is seen in diffuse primary lymphoma of the intestine, but in the terminal ileum.

Fortunately, a definite diagnosis of Whipple's disease can be made by peroral biopsy of the small intestine, which usually shows the histologic changes described above. If laparotomy is performed, examination of a mesenteric lymph node will show the same changes.

Prognosis was formerly hopeless but now, thanks to antibiotics, this has changed. Instead of dying in a state of cachexia, the patient improves dramatically with the aid of antibiotics given over a period of 10 to 12 months. The recommended treatment consists of procaine penicillin, 1,200,000 units/day intramuscularly for 10 days to two weeks, followed by a broad-spectrum antibiotic (e.g., tetracycline, 250 mg orally four times daily) for 10 to 12 months.

Bibliography

Maizel H, Ruffin JM, Dobbins WO: Whipple's disease. *Medicine* 49:175, 1970

Trier JS: Whipple's disease. In *Gastrointestinal Disease* (Sleisenger MH, Fordtran JS, eds), 2nd ed, p 1103. Philadelphia: Saunders, 1978

SUMMARY

Whipple's disease, intestinal lipodystrophy, is a rare condition in which fats and fatty acids are deposited in the lymphatic tissue of the intestine and mesentery. The lamina propria is infiltrated with macrophages and there are large lipoid deposits here and in the peripheral lymph nodes, liver, spleen, heart valves, lungs, kidneys, adrenal glands, bones, and central nervous system. Rod-shaped bacilli are found. Clinically the condition manifests with malabsorption, fever, arthritis, neurologic derangement, diffuse cutaneous pigmentation, and generalized lymphadenopathy. A definite diagnosis can be made by peroral biopsy of the small intestine. Treatment with a good prognosis is 1,200,000 units of procaine penicillin IM for 10 days to two weeks, followed by tetracycline, 250 mg four times daily, for 10 to 12 months.

Scleroderma of the small intestine

46

About half of patients with scleroderma have small intestinal involvement, and half of these have diarrhea or steatorrhea. Intestinal smooth muscle atrophies and the submucosa, muscularis mucosa, and muscular layer become infiltrated with collagen fibers. The diarrhea and steatorrhea are caused by intestinal stasis with bacterial overgrowth, changes in the intestinal wall, lymphatic obstruction, and/or reduction of blood flow.

In addition to diarrhea and steatorrhea, patients usually have dysphagia and pyrosis caused by altered motility of the lower two-thirds of the esophagus and deranged function of the lower esophageal sphincter with esophagitis secondary

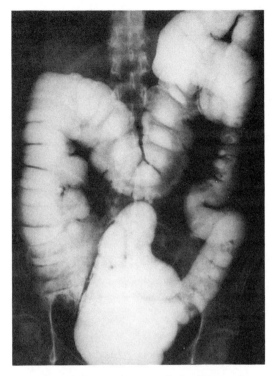

FIGURE 46-1 **Scleroderma of the intestine**
Wide-necked diverticula can be seen in the colon

to gastroesophageal reflux. There are also feelings of fullness, postprandial heaviness, nausea, vomiting, borborygmi, and symptoms of pseudo-obstruction. Some of these patients develop cystic pneumatosis of the intestine and attacks of spontaneous pneumoperitoneum from rupture of the air-filled cysts, which may simulate an acute abdomen. Nearly always they have Raynaud's syndrome and the skin signs of scleroderma. Progressive weakness and weight loss are seen in all these patients.

X-rays are most valuable in making the diagnosis of scleroderma of the intestine. They show a lack of peristalsis in the lower two-thirds of the esophagus, incompetence of the lower esophageal sphincter, dilation of the duodenum, which retains barium for an abnormal length of time, dilation of the intestinal loops with flocculation and segmentation of the barium column, characteristic thickening of the mucosal folds (plicae circulares), slow intestinal passage, and wide-necked pseudodiverticula in the colon, as illustrated in Figure 46-1.

Treatment consists of intermittent courses of broad-spectrum antibiotics, especially tetracycline and ampicillin, elemental diets (Chapter 44), and parenteral solutions of liquids, electrolytes, nutrients, and vitamins. The antibiotics temporarily reduce bacterial overgrowth in the dilated loops of the intestine and consequently control the steatorrhea. In spite of these measures, the disease progresses and the patient finally dies.

Bibliography

Cohen S, Laufer I, Snape WJ, et al: The gastrointestinal manifestations of scleroderma: Pathogenesis and management. *Gastroenterology* 79:155, 1980

Kahn IJ, Jeffries GH, Sleisenger MH: Malabsorption in intestinal scleroderma. Correction by antibiotics. *N Engl J Med* 274:1339, 1966

SUMMARY

About 25 per cent of patients with scleroderma have diarrhea or steatorrhea due to stasis with bacterial overgrowth and changes in the intestinal wall. This is usually accompanied by symptomatic obstruction and reduction of blood flow. Dysphagia, pyrosis, feeling of fullness, nausea and vomiting, borborygmi, and symptoms of pseudo-obstruction may be manifest, as well as progressive weakness and weight loss. X-rays are an important diagnostic modality. Treatment is usually of no avail.

Amyloidosis of the small intestine

47

Amyloidosis is the accumulation of a homogeneous, highly refractile substance with an affinity for Congo red dye. Rokitansky was the first to describe it in 1842 in a case of chronic infection. Ten years later, Virchow gave it the name of amyloid since its staining properties suggested a relationship to starch. It is made up primarily of a well-defined fibril, distinct from extracellular structural proteins, which occurs in two forms. In one form, known as the Ig type, immunoglobulin light chains appear to be the principal protein component; in the other form, called the protein A type, an apparently non-immunoglobulin constituent is the major protein.

Amyloid distribution varies, which explains its multifarious clinical picture. It is deposited especially in the walls of the blood vessels, mainly the small arterioles, as well as in the renal glomeruli, liver, and spleen. It is found adjacent to the basal membrane, and though microscopically it looks amorphous, its fibrillar structure becomes apparent with the electron microscope. The pathologist easily identifies it because of its characteristic staining properties. Iodine stains it brown. If sulfuric acid is added, it turns blue or blue-black. Hematoxylin-eosin stains it red; methyl or cresyl violet produces a metachromatic effect; Congo red imparts a characteristic rosy or red color as well as fluorescence. Amyloid is doubly refractive under polarized light.

Amyloidosis may be physiologic or pathologic. The physiologic type is found very frequently in people over 60 years of age. The deposits are small and probably without clinical significance. Pathologic amyloidosis is classified as primary, secondary, or the amyloidosis of multiple myeloma.

Primary amyloidosis is the most common. It occurs independently of any other disease and affects the mesodermic tissues: the cardiovascular and digestive systems, smooth and striated muscle, and lymph nodes. In some cases it's similar to secondary amyloidosis, as in familial Mediterranean fever. It may be familial. Sometimes it occurs as a diffuse infiltration or localizes in a small area in tumor form.

Secondary amyloidosis occurs in patients with chronic infectious or inflammatory diseases that run a long course. It is seen in 25 per cent of cases of rheumatoid arthritis and in 33 per cent of the lepers at Carville. It is a frequent cause of death in paraplegics who suffer from decubitus ulcers and urinary infections. It has been seen in cases of chronic colitis and enteritis. Extensive deposits of amyloid are found especially in the spleen, liver, kidneys, and adrenal glands. The clinical picture is characterized by nephrotic syndrome, renal insufficiency, hepatomegaly, and splenomegaly.

Amyloidosis occurs in 10 to 20 per cent of cases of multiple myeloma, where it's similar to secondary amyloidosis.

Information is limited regarding malabsorption syndrome from amyloidosis of the small intestine. Herskovic et al examined the charts of 103 patients, 59 of whom had the primary form and 44 the secondary form. Of the 59 with the primary form, five had malabsorption, and of the 44 with the secondary form, only one had malabsorption. The patients with malabsorption had the usual clinical picture: diarrhea, weight loss, weakness, paresthesias, changes in skin sensation, postural hypotension, and steatorrhea. The pathogenesis of the altered intestinal absorption is not clear, but it may be due to destruction of the mucosa by extensive infiltration with amyloid material, poor circulation, and intestinal stasis with bacterial overgrowth.

The best way to make a diagnosis is by biopsy of the rectal mucosa. Material from the free border of one of the valves is best. By means of special staining, diagnosis can be made in 75 per cent of the cases. Sometimes it's possible to make the diagnosis from a biopsy of the small intestine where amyloid deposits are seen in the muscularis mucosae and in the walls of the arteries in the submucosa.

X-rays show nonspecific changes difficult to differentiate from those seen in other malabsorption syndromes.

Although quite rare, amyloidosis should be considered in the differential diagnosis of malabsorption syndromes. Likewise, in all patients with diseases that could give rise to amyloidosis, the appearance of chronic diarrhea and especially of steatorrhea should suggest the possibility of amyloid infiltration into the walls of the intestine.

Bibliography

Battle WM, Rubin MR, Cohen S, et al: Gastrointestinal motility dysfunction in amyloidosis. *N Engl J Med* 301:24, 1979

Gilat T, Spiro HM: Amyloidosis and the gut. *Am J Dig Dis* 13:619, 1968

Herskovic T, Bartholomew LG, Green DA: Amyloidosis and malabsorption syndrome. *Arch Intern Med* 114:629, 1964

SUMMARY

Amyloidosis is the accumulation of a homogeneous, highly refractile fibrillar substance staining a fluorescent rose or red with Congo red. It is deposited in the walls of small arterioles, renal glomeruli, and the liver and spleen. The condition may be physiologic, appearing in those over 60, where it has little significance. Its pathologic forms are primary, secondary, or as part of multiple myeloma. The primary variety is the most common, affecting mesodermic tissue. The secondary variety follows chronic, long-term infectious or inflammatory diseases. It is present in 10 to 20 per cent of those with multiple myeloma. It often causes a malabsorption syndrome. The most certain diagnostic measure is biopsy of the rectum or small intestine.

Intestinal lymphangiectasia

48

One of the final steps in the absorption of fat is its passage into the lymphatics, through which it reaches the bloodstream and finally the tissues. Obviously, disturbances in the lymphatic circulation can lead to steatorrhea.

Obstruction of the lymph vessels and their consequent dilation, lymphangiectasia, can be primary or secondary. Primary lymphangiectasia is probably due to congenital malformation and is evident from infancy. It involves not only the intestinal lymphatics but the whole lymphatic system. Secondary intestinal lymphangiectasia is caused by retroperitoneal fibrosis, retroperitoneal tumors, chronic pancreatitis, lymphomas, intestinal tuberculosis, regional enteritis, radiation enteritis, scleroderma of the intestine, constrictive pericarditis, or congestive heart failure.

The results of this obstructive form, whatever its cause, are steatorrhea and transudation of the lymph, rich in proteins and lymphocytes, into the intestine, from which it is lost in the feces. Clinically, the results are edema from hypoalbuminemia, altered cellular and humoral immunity from the loss of immunoglobulins and lymphocytes, steatorrhea, and malnutrition.

Diagnosis is made by peroral biopsy of the small intestine. Characteristic findings are dilated lymph vessels full of macrophages, which are in turn full of lipids, and distortion of the intestinal villi. Clinical, laboratory, and X-ray studies, including lymphangiography, give information that differentiates the primary form from the secondary form and, if it is secondary, information as to what has caused it.

Treatment of primary lymphangiectasia consists of a completely fat-free diet or substituting medium-chain triglycerides for ordinary fats made up of long-chain triglycerides. These can be absorbed by the portal venous circulation without involving the damaged lymphatic circulation. Results are very good in most cases. Sometimes surgery is indicated to create anastomoses and short circuits to bypass the areas of lymphatic obstruction. When the intestinal lymphangiectasia is secondary, its treatment consists of correcting the primary disease. Here, also, restriction of fats in the diet and substituting medium-chain triglycerides are very helpful.

Bibliography

Herskovic T, Winauer SJ, Goldsmith R, et al: Intestinal lymphangiectasia. *Gastroenterology* 50:849, 1966

Kowlessar OD: Intestinal lymphangiectasia and abetalipoproteinemia. In *Gastrointestinal Disease* (Sleisenger MH, Fordtran JS, eds), 2nd ed, p 1201. Philadelphia: Saunders, 1978

Primary diffuse lymphoma of the small intestine

49

Lymphocytes are abundant in the lamina propria of the small intestine, forming follicles in the mucosa and submucosa and Peyer's patches in the terminal ileum. It's not surprising that lymphomas occur here. Lymphomas frequently affect various parts of the body at the same time, including the bowel. In such cases the term "secondary lymphoma of the small intestine" is frequently employed. Less frequently the neoplasm is restricted to the gut and is called "primary lymphoma of the small intestine." Primary lymphoma may localize in a limited area, occur in multiple foci, or invade a large part of the intestine diffusely. This is the type that gives rise to the malabsorption syndrome.

Primary diffuse lymphoma of the small intestine, known also as Mediterranean lymphoma, is rare except in the Middle East. It is also found in Mexicans and Mexican-Americans. It often affects young adults.

The clinical picture is so similar to that of celiac sprue that this is the diagnosis usually made. Certain differences, however, should impress the alert clinician: anorexia, which contrasts with the normal or even increased appetite of celiac patients; marked hypoproteinemia and edema not only from deficient absorption of nutrients but also from loss of proteins through the intestinal wall; anemia; and, above all, abdominal pain that is sometimes intense in marked contrast to the minimal discomfort of classical celiac sprue. The fever, adenopathy, and hepatosplenomegaly so common in patients with disseminated lymphoma do not occur in patients with primary diffuse lymphoma of the intestine. In any case, a gluten-free diet, no matter how strictly observed, does not change the clinical picture. This definitely rules out celiac sprue.

Laboratory tests do not make the differential diagnosis since the findings are typical of malabsorption syndrome, seen in many diseases. Neither do X-ray studies solve the problem, since they show only the nonspecific changes in the small intestine described in Chapter 20. Sometimes, however, they reveal marked thickening of the folds and walls of the intestine. If this occurs in the terminal ileum, it has some diagnostic value.

When there is lymphomatous infiltration of the mucosa and submucosa of the small intestine, peroral biopsy can make the diagnosis of primary diffuse lymphoma (Chapter 25). Taking specimens from different levels increases the chances of success. One or even several negative biopsies showing merely villous atrophy do not rule out lymphoma.

Some studies indicate that celiac sprue can develop into primary diffuse lymphoma more frequently than would be explained by chance. This happens more often when the patient does not stay on a gluten-free diet. Without denying this possibility, it's wise to consider that the diffuse lymphoma could have existed from the beginning, simulating celiac sprue.

Sometimes a diagnosis is impossible. Some cases of primary diffuse lymphoma show an immunoglobulin (IgA type) devoid of light chains and characteristically composed of heavy chains of the alpha-1 subclass.

The prognosis is poor. Treatment consists only of maintaining the patient's nutritional state by means of parenteral feedings. Surgery is contraindicated because the process is so extensive. Radiotherapy and chemotherapy have not given good results.

Bibliography

Eidelman S, Parkins RA, Rubin CE: Abdominal lymphoma presenting as malabsorption. *Medicine* 45:111, 1966

Gray GM, Rosenberg SA, Cooper AD, et al: Lymphomas involving the gastrointestinal tract. *Gastroenterology* 82:143, 1982

Seligmann M: Immunochemical, clinical and pathological features of alpha-chain disease. *Arch Intern Med* 135:78, 1975

Zarrabi MH, Rosner F: Middle Eastern intestinal lymphoma: Report of a case and review of the literature *Am J Med Sci* 272:101, 1976

SUMMARY

Primary lymphoma may localize in one or multiple areas or be diffuse. The latter variety is known as Mediterranean lymphoma. Clinically this condition is similar to celiac sprue except for anorexia, hypoproteinemia, anemia, and severe abdominal pain. Most important in differentiating it from celiac sprue is its lack of response to a gluten-free diet. The diagnosis is difficult, as laboratory tests or X-rays are not pathognomonic. Where there is infiltration of the mucosa and submucosa, peroral biopsy may be of great help. The prognosis is poor. Treatment is purely supportive.

Immunodeficiency and malabsorption

50

Malabsorption may occur in primary acquired agammaglobulinemia, in selective deficiency of IgA, and in deficiency of IgA and IgM. The pathogenesis of malabsorption in these syndromes is not well understood. Bacterial overgrowth, favored by the immunodeficiency, has been considered. Bacterial counts support this theory.

Primary acquired agammaglobulinemia

Primary acquired agammaglobulinemia is characterized by extremely low levels of all the immunoglobulins in the blood. The onset may be at any age, with recurrent bacterial infections, rheumatoid arthritis, and other autoimmune phenomena in about 30 per cent of the cases. Malignant lymphoreticular tumors, hyperplasia of lymphatic tissue, and intestinal symptoms also occur.

Intestinal symptoms are found in 20 to 50 per cent according to various reports and consist of diarrhea or frank malabsorption. In malabsorption, the symptoms, laboratory findings, and X-rays are the same as in celiac sprue but peroral biopsy findings are different. The villi do not atrophy and plasma cells do not infiltrate the lamina propria. Most of these patients have hyperplasia of the intestinal lymphoid tissue, which may cause a protein-losing gastroenteropathy. This makes the hypogammaglobulinemia worse. The lymphoid hyperplasia is seen on X-rays as numerous small circular filling defects similar to those seen in IgA and IgM deficiencies. The frequency with which these patients suffer infestations with *Giardia lamblia* is impressive. This parasite may be seen in intestinal biopsies.

Various treatments have been tried: periodic injections of commercial gamma globulin, infusions of fresh plasma, broad-spectrum antibiotics, medication against *G. lamblia,* gluten-free diet, and cholestyramine. Regular injections of commercial gamma globulin are undoubtedly useful in preventing bacterial infections, especially if the gamma globulin in the serum is maintained at a level above 200 mg/100 ml. This, however, does not control the intestinal symptoms since commercial gamma globulin does not contain IgA. Fresh plasma does contain IgA and is therefore more beneficial. Broad-spectrum antibiotics are of some value, which supports the theory that malabsorption is caused by bacterial overgrowth. Cholestyramine is sometimes helpful. It takes up bile acids, which would otherwise be changed by bacterial action and cause diarrhea.

Deficiency of IgA causes symptoms as well as physiologic and structural changes very similar to those seen in celiac sprue. IgA is absent or greatly decreased not only in the blood serum but also in all exocrine secretions, including digestive secretions. Peroral biopsy of the small intestine shows both the abnormalities of celiac sprue and a marked reduction or absence in the lamina propria of the plasma cells that synthesize IgA. These patients improve on a gluten-free diet. It's evident, however, that they do not have celiac sprue because in celiac sprue the blood levels of IgA are normal and even increased and plasma cells that secrete this immunoglobulin abound in the lamina propria of the intestine.

Dysgammaglobulinemia

Among the less common causes of malabsorption is dysgammaglobulinemia, so called because there are disproportionate reductions in serum IgA and IgM. Very frequently these patients are parasitized by *G. lamblia.* X-ray studies of the small intestine show characteristic abnormalities that consist of nodules 1 to 3 mm in diameter uniformly distributed all along the small intestine and sometimes in the right colon. The nodules are lymphatic follicles with large germinal centers located in the lamina propria. The intestinal villi and even the epithelial cells look normal under the microscope; there is no atrophy. This definitely separates dysgammaglobulinemic patients from those who have acquired hypogammaglobulinemia and a spruelike syndrome but with atrophied jejunal mucosa.

In patients with dysgammaglobulinemia the intestinal biopsy also shows reduction in plasma cells, the source of IgA, so important in protecting the intestine and other mucous surfaces from infection. It's logical to suppose that IgA is decreased in intestinal secretions, thus permitting bacterial overgrowth and diarrhea. Improvement with antibiotics supports this view. Again, parenteral treatment with commercial gamma globulin is not effective because it doesn't contain IgA. Plasma, however, does contain IgA and is effective treatment. A case is on record in which the patient had selective deficiency of IgA from the age of 6 months; this patient improved considerably with monthly injections of fresh plasma.

Bibliography

Crabbé PA, Hermans JF: Selective IgA deficiency with steatorrhea: A new syndrome. *Am J Med* 42:319, 1967

Doe WF: An overview of intestinal immunity and malabsorption. *Am J Med* 67:1077, 1979

Hermans PE, Huizenga KA, Hoffman H, et al: Dysgammaglobulinemia associated with nodular lymphoid hyperplasia of the small intestine. *Am J Med* 40:78, 1966

Hersh T, Floch M, Binder HJ, et al: Disturbance of the jejunal and colonic bacterial flora in immunoglobulin deficiencies. *Am J Clin Nutr* 23:1595, 1970

Webster AD: The gut and immunodeficiency disorders. *Clin Gastroenterol* 5:323, 1976

SUMMARY

Although not all immunodeficiencies result in malabsorption, it does occur in a number of them. Primary acquired agammaglobulinemia at any age is accompanied by recurrent bacterial infection and autoimmune syndromes such as rheumatoid arthritis. Giardiasis is also common. Diarrhea occurs if the intestine is involved. Peroral biopsy differentiates primary acquired agammaglobulinemia from celiac sprue. The best treatment is fresh plasma and broad-spectrum antibiotics.

Deficiency of IgA (dysgammaglobulinemia, single) causes a celiac sprue-like syndrome and improvement follows a gluten-free diet. In celiac sprue, however, IgA serum levels are normal.

In multiple dysgammaglobulinemia, both IgA and IgM levels are below normal. Here X-ray and peroral biopsy are important diagnostic modalities. Giardiasis and bacterial overgrowth are common. Treatment is plasma and broad-spectrum antibiotics.

Carcinoid tumors

51

Carcinoids are tumors of entero-chromaffin cells that appear occasionally in the digestive tract, bronchi, and ovaries. They occur most often in the appendix, then, in decreasing frequency, in the terminal ileum, rectum, colon, stomach, gallbladder, pancreas, Meckel's diverticulum, bronchi, and ovaries. They are small, 1 to 3 cm, and occur singly more often than in groups. They are called carcinoids because they were once erroneously supposed to be benign, in spite of their carcinoma-like appearance. It is now known that they are malignant, although their existence is compatible with long life even in the presence of metastasis. The most malignant carcinoid is found in the terminal ileum, from which it metastasizes to the liver, regional lymph nodes, bones, and lungs. Carcinoids in the appendix rarely metastasize but may cause acute appendicitis because of obstruction, necessitating surgical removal. Histologic examination of the tissue makes the diagnosis.

Carcinoid tumors secrete biologically active substances giving rise to the "carcinoid syndrome." The symptoms are diarrhea, hot flashes, cyanosis, telangiectasis, asthma, and involvement of the valves in the right chambers of the heart. The substances responsible for these symptoms are serotonin (5-hydroxytryptamine), histamine, bradykinin, ectopic ACTH, and an unidentified substance thought to cause the hot flashes.

The diarrhea is caused by serotonin, which has a marked stimulating effect on peristalsis. It's usually explosive and liquid, accompanied by much borborygmi and cramping, flatulence, nausea, and vomiting. Sometimes it is chronic and constant and occasionally it gives rise to the malabsorption syndrome. The hot flashes affect the face, neck, upper part of the thorax, and superior extremities. They are repetitive and paroxysmal, lasting a few minutes and causing blushing accompanied by a burning sensation followed first by cyanosis and then by pallor. They may be accompanied by dyspnea or frank asthmatic wheezing. Emotional tension, physical exercise, or ingestion of alcoholic beverages and food precipitates attacks.

Physical examination reveals telangiectasis on the face and the systolic ejection murmur of pulmonary stenosis. The valvular lesion is caused by deposits of fibrous tissue. High blood concentrations of serotonin are considered responsible.

The syndrome occurs only when the serotonin and other substances reach the general circulation. This happens when the tumors are located outside the region of the portal vein or when there is a metastasis to the liver, enabling the carcinoid secretions to reach the hepatic veins and escape the action of the hepatic inactivating enzymes.

Diarrhea accompanied by one or more symptoms of the carcinoid syndrome suggests the diagnosis. The urinary excretion of excessive amounts of 5-hydroxyindoleacetic acid, a metabolite of serotonin, establishes the diagnosis. Nine milligrams per day is the maximum normal amount excreted, but only amounts over 25 mg/day are diagnostic since excretion of 9 to 25 mg/day may be due to other intestinal diseases. Some foods, especially bananas and nuts, are very rich in serotonin and should be eliminated from the diet before the test.

Another test for serotonin is the intravenous injection of 1 μg of epinephrine. The epinephrine stimulates the liberation of secretions that cause the hot flashes, as well as serotonin. The hot flashes appear within 90 seconds in a positive test. If the test is negative, increasing amounts of epinephrine up to 10 μg may be tried.

Carcinoids produce mesenteric fibrosis and angulation of the intestinal loops, giving the characteristic X-ray picture described in Chapter 20.

The treatment may be surgical, with resection of the primary tumor in an ovary or in one bronchus, or partial hepatectomy when this is feasible, to remove metastatic lesions. Some patients have had good results from the regional arterial infusion of 5-fluorouracil. Diarrhea and other symptoms may be alleviated by medications that modify the action of the chemical mediators found in the carcinoid secretions, such as antagonists of serotonin—methysergide (Sansert) and cyproheptadine (Periactin); that block the synthesis of serotonin—p-chlorophenylalanine; or that relieve the hot flashes and the diarrhea—phenothiazines and corticosteroids. Diarrhea is best controlled with cyproheptadine and methysergide, but these medicines have undesirable side effects, such as drowsiness (cyproheptadine) and dangerous retroperitoneal fibrosis (methysergide).

Bibliography

Kowlessar OD: The carcinoid syndrome. In *Gastrointestinal Disease* (Sleisenger MH, Fordtran JS, eds), 2nd ed, p 1190. Philadelphia: Saunders, 1978

Sjoderma R, Melmon KL: The carcinoid spectrum. *Gastroenterology* 47:104, 1964

Welch JP, Malt RA: Management of carcinoid tumors of the gastrointestinal tract. *Surg Gynecol Obstet* 145:223, 1977

SUMMARY

Carcinoids are small malignant tumors, single or multiple, that may appear in the gastrointestinal tract, especially in the appendix, then the terminal ileum, rectum, colon, stomach, gallbladder, pancreas, and Meckel's diverticulum, in order of frequency. These tumors are compatible with long life although they do metastasize. They secrete serotonin, histamine, bradykinin, ACTH, and an unidentified substance producing the "carcinoid syndrome" of diarrhea, hot flashes, cyanosis, telangiectasis, asthma, and involvement of the right chambers of the heart. Occasionally malabsorption occurs. The diagnosis is made via urinary excretion of large amounts of 5-hydroxyindoleacetic acid. Treatment may be surgery or regional arterial infusion of 5-fluorouracil. Diarrhea is relieved by serotonin antagonists such as cyproheptadine (Periactin) or methysergide (Sansert).

Syndrome of watery diarrhea, hypochlorhydria, and hypokalemia

52

In 1958, Verner and Morrison described a syndrome which bears their names, Verner-Morrison syndrome, and is also known as "pancreatic cholera" and the "watery diarrhea, hypochlorhydria, and hypokalemia syndrome" (WDHH). Chronic liquid diarrhea so copious that it resembles cholera is typical. The patient may pass 6 liters and even up to 9 liters of liquid stools during a period of 24 hours. The patient experiences no pain or tenesmus with defecation. The stool looks like weak tea and is free of mucus, blood, and food residues. The electrolyte content of the stool, especially that of potassium, is very high; 300 mEq or more of potassium are lost daily.

Patients with WDHH syndrome suffer acute dehydration and prostration. The outstanding laboratory finding is hypokalemia, which can be corrected only by giving large quantities of potassium. Other laboratory findings are gastric hypochlorhydria, hypercalcemia, hypomagnesemia, and a diabetic glucose tolerance curve. Some of these patients have hot flashes caused by cutaneous vasodilation in the upper part of the body.

Most patients with WDHH have benign and malignant tumors of non-beta islet cells of the pancreas. Others have hyperplasia of these same delta cells of the pancreas, and still others, bronchogenic carcinomas. One patient had pheochromocytoma, and another had ganglioneuroblastoma of the adrenal gland. Surgical removal of the tumor—total pancreatectomy in the case of diffuse hyperplasia of the delta cells—and chemotherapy with streptozocin in cases with metastases have been curative. Corticosteroids, indomethacin (Indocin), and lithium carbonate may reduce or abolish the diarrhea.

In many but not all cases, production of the digestive hormone VIP (vasoactive intestinal polypeptide) occurs. The pharmacologic properties of this polypeptide explain the altered pathophysiology. This hormone stimulates the intestinal secretion of water and electrolytes, inhibits the secretion of hydrochloric acid, raises the level of serum calcium, produces hyperglycemia by increasing glycogenolysis in the liver, and dilates the peripheral arterioles. Radioimmunoassay has shown high levels of VIP in the blood in many of these patients, in extracts from the tumors, and in the culture medium containing cells from a pancreatic adenoma causing the disease. Besides VIP, one or more substances such as prostaglandin E must be implicated in some patients with WDHH syndrome.

Suspect this disease in all patients with choleriform diarrhea that is chronic, noninfectious, and resistant to symptomatic treatment, especially if there is also hypokalemia. Where this is so, the other symptoms of the disease should be looked for and blood samples sent to the proper laboratory for VIP testing. A celiac arteriogram, hepatic and pancreatic scans, and chest X-rays help locate many of these tumors.

Diagnosis based on clinical and laboratory findings, especially high blood levels of VIP, justifies surgical exploration
if the tumor has not yet been located. Laparotomy may be the
only way to discover pancreatic and extrapancreatic tumors, especially hyperplastic processes of the pancreas.

Bibliography

Jaffe BM, Condon S: Prostaglandins E and F in endocrine diarrheagenic
    syndromes. *Ann Surg* 184:516, 1976

Jaffe BM, Kopen DF, DeSchryver-Kecskemeti K, et al: Indomethacin-
    responsive pancreatic cholera. *N Engl J Med* 297:817, 1977

Kahn CR, Levy AG, Gardner JD, et al: Pancreatic cholera: Beneficial ef-
    fects of treatment with streptozotocin. *N Engl J Med* 292:941, 1975

Said SI, Faloona GD: Elevated plasma and tissue levels of vasoactive intes-
    tinal polypeptide in the watery diarrhea syndrome due to pancreatic,
    bronchogenic and other tumors. *N Engl J Med* 293:155, 1975

Verner JV, Morrison AB: Islet cell tumor and a syndrome of refractory
    watery diarrhea and hypokalemia. *Am J Med* 25:374, 1958

SUMMARY

This syndrome (WDHH) is also called the Verner-Morrison
syndrome or pancreatic cholera. Patients suffer copious liquid diarrhea with loss of large amounts of potassium. Laboratory findings also show gastric hypochlorhydria,
hypercalcemia, hypomagnesemia, and a diabetic glucose
tolerance curve. Acute dehydration and prostration are the
major symptoms. Tumors of the pancreatic cells are the
usual cause, and often there is production of vasoactive intestinal polypeptide. If the laboratory tests do not localize
the tumor(s), laparotomy is in order.

Gastric surgery, malabsorption, and diarrhea

53

Partial gastrectomy of whatever type results in diarrhea and deficient intestinal absorption in quite a few cases. Data vary greatly from author to author, but all agree that the symptoms are usually mild and temporary except in about 2 per cent of cases. These few patients lose weight and cannot gain it back. They have steatorrhea, creatorrhea, and anemia, usually hypochromic and rarely macrocytic. The diarrhea is of osmotic origin, which was explained in Chapter 2.

Etiology

Rapid transit of the intestinal contents is considered to be the cause of the malabsorption, since the food does not remain in contact with the intestinal mucosa long enough to be properly absorbed. Nevertheless, patients with steatorrhea excrete the same amount of fecal fat whether they have diarrhea or have had their diarrhea controlled by medication. Steatorrhea is less frequent and severe following gastrectomy with Billroth I anastomosis than with Billroth II, which indicates that when food does not pass through the duodenum the pancreas is not stimulated and functional pancreatic insufficiency results. Insufficiency of bile secretion could also result. Pancreatic and biliary secretions normally reach the duodenum simultaneously with food, resulting in complete mixing, emulsification, and hydrolysis of fats. Following gastrectomy or gastroenterostomy, however, this synchrony is lost. Food arrives prematurely and is moved along the intestine without the action of pancreatic enzymes and bile salts. There is no doubt that this explains the steatorrhea and creatorrhea in some cases, since with pancreatic supplements the excretion of fats and proteins in the stool has been observed to diminish and these patients soon begin to gain weight.

It has been suggested that the afferent loop acts as a blind loop harboring bacteria in large numbers. The bacterial overgrowth results in steatorrhea and competitive consumption of vitamin B_{12}. In some patients the steatorrhea and absorption of vitamin B_{12} have improved with antibiotics.

Some patients may have a primary, latent, or subclinical defect in intestinal absorption made worse by the resection of part of the stomach.

It is not necessary to have undergone a partial gastrectomy with anastomosis to the intestine to develop diarrhea and malabsorption. These symptoms may occur after vagotomy or pyloroplasty. Sixty per cent of such patients have mild transitory diarrhea, but in 5 per cent it becomes a serious problem. Its cause is not understood, but bacterial overgrowth secondary to hypochlorhydria and decreased peristalsis following vagotomy may be factors. Since broad-spectrum antibiotics and cholinergics such as bethanechol (Urecholine) are beneficial, this may be the explanation. On the other hand, some patients improve with the very opposite treatment, such as antidiarrheal medication that slows peristalsis or surgical implantation of antiperistaltic loops.

Surgical prevention

In an effort to overcome these effects of complete vagotomy, a selective and a superselective vagotomy have been devised. Selective vagotomy consists of cutting only the part of the nerve that goes to the stomach and leaving the celiac and hepatic branches intact. Superselective vagotomy spares the branches to the gastric antrum and sections only those that innervate the body of the stomach and therefore the parietal cells responsible for secretion of acid. In this way, gastric emptying continues to take place normally. These operations are effective in preventing diarrhea.

Treatment

The medical treatment of diarrhea and malabsorption in patients who have had gastric surgery is easy in mild cases and extremely difficult in severe ones. Ideally, an exact diagnosis of the pathophysiology involved is necessary. This includes X-rays or radioisotope scanning for evaluation of gastric emptying, measurement of exocrine pancreatic secretion, measurement of the aerobic and anaerobic flora in the upper intestine, and evaluation of the activity of abnormal flora in consuming D-xylose and vitamin B_{12}. With this information, you can determine whether the patient needs pancreatic enzymes and bile salts, antibiotics, or surgery to correct the rapid gastric emptying, stasis in the afferent loop, or excessive peristalsis.

In practice, an empirical course is usually decided on: The rapid gastric emptying is prevented by a dry diet and frequent small meals free of mono- and oligosaccharides because of their high osmolarity. If necessary, the patient should lie down while eating or immediately after. The next step consists of giving pancreatic extracts and in some cases bile salts in doses sufficient to control the steatorrhea partially or completely: 1 or 2 gm of pancreatic extract before and after each meal or 1 to 2 gm every two or three hours during the day. If this treatment is not sufficient, 1 to 2 gm/day of tetracycline or some other broad-spectrum antibiotic is given for one or two weeks. Since improvement with antibiotics is temporary, they must be given intermittently, with dosage and length of the treatment adjusted to the individual case. These methods are usually successful. If not, elemental diets, medium-chain triglycerides, parenteral alimentation, and surgery may be indicated (see Chapter 44).

In patients whose malabsorption is caused by failure of pancreatic enzymes and bile salts to act on food before it reaches the intestine, these secretions can be stimulated half an hour before meals with a simple procedure recommended years ago by Avery Jones: Have the patient take a slice of bread and butter and a glass of orange juice half an hour before meals.

Bibliography

Craft IL, Venobles CW: Antiperistaltic segment of jejunum for persistent diarrhea following vagotomy. *Ann Surg* 167:282, 1968

Lund G: The mechanism of post-gastrectomy malabsorption. *Gastroenterology* 42:637, 1962

SUMMARY

Partial gastrectomy may result in diarrhea and deficient absorption. Some patients lose weight and have steatorrhea, creatorrhea, and anemia. This may occur after vagotomy or pyloroplasty. Bacterial overgrowth secondary to hypochlorhydria and diminished peristalsis may be a factor. Variations of vagotomy have been devised that prevent these complications. Proper treatment depends upon exact etiology. Empirical treatment consists of a dry diet, frequent small meals free of mono- and oligosaccharides (the patient should lie down while eating or immediately thereafter), pancreatic extracts with or without bile salts, and one or two weeks of tetracycline.

Bacterial overgrowth syndrome

54

The normal stomach and jejunum contain comparatively few bacteria, the majority of which are gram-positive aerobic or facultative anaerobic organisms, especially enterococci and lactobacilli. Their concentration is 10 to 10^4/ml of duodenal fluid. It increases up to 10^5 to 10^8/ml in the distal portion of the ileum, where gram-negative organisms, especially coliforms and *Bacteroides,* also occur. Once the ileocecal valve is passed, the concentration rises sharply in the colon to 10^9 to 10^{11}/ml, with 1,000 anaerobes for every aerobe. The most important colonic species are *Bacteroides, Clostridium,* and anaerobic lactobacilli. The concentration expelled in the feces is 10 to 100 times that in the colon.

Normal intestinal flora

At birth the digestive tract is sterile. Bacteria reach it via food, and in three to four weeks the bacterial concentration becomes constant and characteristic for each individual throughout the years, unaffected by changes in diet or place of abode unless these changes are very great. Why the upper parts of the digestive tract are so free from bacteria may be explained by the hydrochloric acid in the stomach, the antiseptic action of bile, peristalsis of the stomach, duodenum, and jejunum, the antibacterial action of secretory IgA, and the mechanical barrier of the ileocecal valve.

The various species of bacteria live in ecologic equilibrium not only among themselves but with the host. However, the bacteria compete for nutrients. In addition there are toxic metabolites, alterations in pH and oxidation-reduction potential, synthesis of growth factors, sharing of enzymes, and transmission of factors (plasmids) resistant to antibiotics. Some bacteria produce antibiotic compounds called colicins, and also medium-chain fatty acids that have the ability to destroy pathogenic bacteria such as *Salmonella typhi*. Thus the indiscriminate administration of antibiotics may do harm by destroying the indigenous flora and upsetting the ecologic equilibrium.

The bacterial population of the intestine affects its structure and function. Animals whose gut has been maintained sterile from birth have longer villi in the intestinal walls than normal animals and they have less cellular infiltration, few lymphocytes and reticuloendothelial cells, few mitoses in the crypt cells, very few Peyer's patches, and no plasma cells. In contrast, normal animals and humans show inflammatory characteristics that can be called "physiologic inflammation." Likewise the concentration of immunoglobulins is very low in the blood of germfree animals but ascends to normal values when the intestine acquires a normal flora.

In the normal individual, intestinal bacteria act on carbohydrates, proteins, and fats. They ferment the carbohydrates, especially the disaccharides if ingested in excess or if disaccharidase deficiency has prevented them from being broken down and absorbed. This fermentation produces short-chain organic acids, hydrogen, and carbon dioxide. The action of the bacteria on proteins converts tryptophan into indole, urea and glycine into ammonia, and methionine into sulfuric acid and dimethyl sulfate. The fats are changed into hydroxylated acids. Bacteria act on sterols and steroids, including bile salts, which they break down and dehydroxylate, and on bilirubin, which after reduction is converted into stercobilinogens (urobilinogens). Bacteria consume vitamin B_{12}, depriving the host of this vitamin and favoring the development of megaloblastosis. They synthesize vitamin K and produce, but also consume, folates.

Pathogenesis of malabsorption

Malabsorption is essentially due to the invasion of the upper parts of the digestive tract by flora that normally inhabit the colon. This happens when there is interference with one or more of the factors that control the sterility of the upper segments. Clinical experience indicates that the most important of these is intestinal stasis and the next in importance is achlorhydria. The syndrome therefore occurs in individuals with blind loops, diverticula, stenosis, fistulae, defective emptying of the afferent loop, partial gastrectomy, vagotomy, autonomic diabetic neuropathy, intestinal scleroderma, amyloidosis, diffuse primary lymphoma, or regional enteritis. In diffuse primary lymphoma the syndrome develops when parts of the intestine become stenosed with resultant stasis. In many of these cases a flora similar to what is normally limited to the colon develops in the upper part of the intestine. The bacterial count reaches $10^{10}/$ ml. As a consequence vitamin B_{12} is partially consumed and abnormal breakdown and dehydroxylation of bile salts interferes with the formation of micelles, and consequently with the absorption of fats. The abnormal bile salts also cause diarrhea by direct action on the colon.

Diagnosis

The diagnosis of malabsorption syndrome should be considered in all patients who have chronic diarrhea or steatorrhea combined with the predisposing factors already mentioned. The diagnosis is established when concentrations of bacteria are found in excess of 10^5/ml from cultures of material aspirated from the duodenum or jejunum. Unfortunately, this direct method of diagnosis is not possible in most clinical laboratories. Indirect methods are more commonly used. One of these is the administration of broad-spectrum antibiotics. A positive result consists of definite clinical improvement with corresponding improvement in the blood levels of carotene and in the D-xylose and vitamin B_{12} absorption tests. This improvement is temporary.

Another simple method is quantitative determination of urinary indican. Indican, the potassium salt of indoxyl sulfate, results from bacterial action on tryptophan that releases its side chain and converts it to indole, which is absorbed, hydroxylated, and esterified in the liver and eliminated by the kidneys as indican. Indicanuria in excess of 100 mg/24 hours suggests bacterial overgrowth.

Tests of absorption of D-xylose and radioactive vitamin B_{12} give more exact results. Deficient absorption of D-xylose corrected by the administration of antibiotics indicates bacterial overgrowth in the jejunum. Deficient absorption of vitamin B_{12} not corrected by the addition of intrinsic factor but corrected by antibiotics also indicates bacterial overgrowth.

Several breath test techniques are of value in the diagnosis of the bacterial overgrowth syndrome. Their common principle is continuous or periodic measurement in the breath of the specific bacterial metabolite of a substrate ingested by the patient. The most commonly used test is the bile acid breath test, which detects bacterial cleavage of the amide bond linking labeled glycine with cholic acid.

Treatment

Unfortunately, the beneficial effects of antibiotics are temporary. When they are discontinued, the bacteria grow back and the symptoms return. More permanent results can be obtained only by correcting the conditions that predispose to bacterial overgrowth. The most important of these is in-

TABLE 54-1

Causes of bacterial overgrowth

Decrease in gastric acid secretion
Pernicious anemia
Chronic gastritis
Postgastrectomy and vagotomy syndromes

Altered intestinal motility
Diabetes mellitus
Scleroderma
Amyloidosis
Celiac sprue
Intestinal pseudo-obstruction

Obstruction of the small intestine
Stenosis
Regional enteritis

Immunoglobulin deficiency
Hypogammaglobulinemia
IgA deficiency
IgA and IgM deficiency (dysgammaglobulinemia
   with lymphoid nodular hyperplasia of the intestine)

Removal of the ileocecal valve
Internal enteric fistulae
Surgical resections
Surgical short circuits

testinal stasis. Surgery may be effective in correcting blind loops, fistulae, and subocclusive conditions and may improve the functioning of the afferent loop in patients who have had gastroenteroanastomosis of the Billroth II type. When the primary process is a peristaltic defect, as in diabetic neuropathy or scleroderma, surgery has nothing to offer and the only treatment available is intermittent therapy with tetracyclines or other broad-spectrum antibiotics.

Table 54-1 lists the different causes of bacterial overgrowth in the intestine.

Bibliography

Donaldson RM: Malabsorption in the blind loop syndrome. *Gastroenterology* 48:388, 1965

Hepner GW: Breath tests in gastroenterology. *Adv Intern Med* 23:25, 1978

Isaacs PE, Young SK: The contaminated small bowel syndrome. *Am J Med* 67:1049, 1979

SUMMARY

The bacterial overgrowth syndrome results in malabsorption due to invasion of the upper gastrointestinal tract by flora that normally inhabit the colon. This is most often due to intestinal stasis and achlorhydria. The diagnosis is made when bacterial concentrations above 10^5/ml are found in cultures from duodenal or jejunal aspirates. Other tests of some value are indicanuria over 100 mg/24 hours; deficient D-xylose absorption, and deficient radioactive vitamin B_{12} absorption corrected by antibiotics. The effects of antibiotic therapy are temporary. Surgery may be necessary to correct the cause of intestinal stasis.

Pancreatic insufficiency

55

The external pancreatic secretions amount to approximately 1
liter daily and contain water, bicarbonate and other electrolytes, and the enzymes amylase, lipase, trypsin, chymo-
trypsins A and B, ribonuclease, deoxyribonuclease, phospholipase A, elastase, collagenase, and leucine amino-
peptidase. These enzymes are essential to the digestion of
carbohydrates, fats, and proteins.

Pancreatic function

The pancreatic phase of digestion takes place as follows:
Stimulation by the vagus nerve liberates acetylcholine, dis-

tention of the gastric antrum stimulates the G cells of the
stomach to secrete gastrin, and the food that reaches the duodenum stimulates the secretion of cholecystokinin-pancreozymin (CCK-PZ). Acetylcholine, gastrin, and CCK-PZ acti-
vate receptors in the external membranes of the pancreatic
cells, and these secrete the pancreatic enzymes, many of
which occur as proenzymes. The pancreatic and biliary secretions reach the duodenum, where the proenzymes are ac-
tivated and changed into enzymes by enterokinase and calcium ions. When the pH, the concentration of biliary acids,
and electrolytes are optimal, the enzymes act on their food
substrates and convert them into oligosaccharides, fatty
acids, monoglycerides, amino acids, oligopeptides, and
other relatively small molecules (see Chapters 4, 5, and 6).
An excess of proteolytic enzymes and biliary acids inhibits
the secretion of CCK-PZ and thus suppresses pancreatic
secretion.

Many clinical and experimental studies have shown that
the pancreas, as a gland of external secretion, has great re-
serve powers. In inflammatory processes such as pancreatitis, neoplastic processes such as carcinoma, degenerative
diseases such as cystic fibrosis, severe malnutrition, or obstruction from lithiasis or stenosis of the pancreatic ducts,
the amounts of lipase and trypsin must be reduced by 90 per
cent to produce steatorrhea and creatorrhea, respectively.
This is the reason why pancreatic insufficiency appears so
late in the course of the diseases mentioned.

Diagnosis of insufficiency

The most important symptom in patients who have exocrine
pancreatic insufficiency is steatorrhea (see Chapter 12).
Sometimes steatorrhea is so severe that oil leaks from the
anus. The patients lose weight and show signs of deficiency
of the fat-soluble vitamins, i.e., osteomalacia and hemorrhage with a prolonged prothrombin time.

The differential diagnosis of pancreatic steatorrhea is discussed in Chapter 22. Simple microscopic examination of
emulsified feces shows many fibers of undigested meat; if
Sudan IV is added, many fat droplets are seen. Tests for ab-

sorption of D-xylose, X-rays of the small intestine, and peroral biopsy of the jejunum are normal in patients who have steatorrhea from pancreatic insufficiency.

The best method for measuring the exocrine functional capacity of the pancreas is by means of the secretin test. This is done by passing a double Dreiling tube to aspirate simultaneously and separately the gastric and pancreatic secretions; this is done under the fluoroscope. Two clinical units per kilogram of secretin are given intravenously, and pancreatic juice is collected four times at 20-minute intervals. Its volume and concentration of bicarbonate are then measured.

In chronic pancreatitis, the volume is normal but the bicarbonate is decreased. In obstruction of the pancreatic ducts, only the volume but not the concentration of bicarbonate is decreased. Normal values are 1.8 ml of pancreatic juice per kilogram of body weight per hour; the maximum normal concentration of bicarbonate is 82 mEq/liter, and the minimum normal volume of bicarbonate is 6.2 mEq/hour. Given together, secretin and CCK augment each other's actions, but carefully designed studies on interactions between the two hormones on pancreatic secretion in humans have not been undertaken. In general, combinations of secretin and CCK produce volume, bicarbonate, and enzyme outputs that exceed rates of secretion expected from the sum of responses to similar doses of each agent alone (potentiation).

Other procedures of proved value in the diagnosis of pancreatic diseases are flat films of the abdomen, which may show calcifications characteristic of some cases of chronic pancreatitis; upper gastrointestinal X-rays supplemented with hypotonic duodenography, which may show evidence of extrinsic compression of inflammatory, cystic, or tumoral origin; retrograde endoscopic pancreatography; ultrasonography; computed axial tomography; and selective arteriography.

Treatment

The treatment of exocrine pancreatic insufficiency consists of restriction of fat in the diet and of oral doses of potent pancreatic extracts, 10 to 20 gm/day. Two grams or more may be given before and after meals or at regular intervals every two to three hours. Failure of standard oral pancreatic enzyme replacement therapy is due to acidic and peptic inactivation of ingested enzymes. Supplemental cimetidine has proven beneficial in such cases.

Bibliography

Dreiling DA, Janowitz HD, Perrier CV: *Pancreatic Inflammatory Disease.* New York: Hoeber-Harper & Row, 1964

Regan PT, Malagelada JR, Dimagno EP, et al: Rationale for the use of cimetidine in pancreatic insufficiency. *Mayo Clin Proc* 53:79, 1978

SUMMARY

Pancreatic exocrine secretion is large in volume and persistent in the face of pancreatic disease. Insufficiency appears late in the course of such disease. The most important symptom is steatorrhea that may become very severe. The secretin test is the best means of measuring pancreatic exocrine function. Other diagnostic measures of value are flat films of the abdomen, upper gastrointestinal studies with hypotonic duodenography, retrograde endoscopic pancreatography, CT scan, and selective arteriography. Treatment consists of a low-fat diet, pancreatic extract, and occasionally cimetidine.

Functional disturbances of the colon

56

The patient seen most frequently by gastroenterologists is one who complains of a combination of symptoms indicating that the physiology of the colon is altered. Nevertheless, carefully performed clinical, laboratory, endoscopic, and X-ray studies do not indicate any organic lesion in the colon. The conclusion is that the patient is suffering from functional alterations of the colon, dyssynergy of the colon, mucomembranous colitis, spastic colon, mucous colitis, spasmomyxorrhea, spastic constipation, functional diarrhea, functional enterocolopathy, unstable colon, vegetative neurosis, colonic neurosis, adaptive colitis, or irritable colon. The multiplicity of terms reflects the confusion that exists

ists regarding the etiology, pathogenesis, physiopathology, and essential clinical picture of the syndrome and indicates the individual preferences and prejudices of each author. None of the names is completely adequate. All can be severely criticized. The most popular is not well founded—i.e., irritable colon. At any rate, when faced with a patient who has impaired function of the colon, it's more important to understand the "why" and the "how" of his symptoms than to give a name to this abstraction that is called a "disease."

Symptomatology

The disturbance is more common in women than in men and may appear at any age. Most frequently, however, it occurs in young adults. If the onset is after 50 years of age, functional origin should be doubted.

The cardinal symptoms are abdominal pain, meteorism, constipation, diarrhea, small stools, sensation of incomplete defecation, and mucus in the stools. These symptoms may occur singly or in any combination. They may be continuous or intermittent, with exacerbations and remissions over a period of weeks, months, or years.

The pain is usually in the lower half of the abdomen or localized to one of the lower quadrants, but it may occur in the epigastric area or in one of the upper quadrants. The pain is usually of two types. The first is constant, and is described by the patient as a feeling of distention or heaviness. It is made worse by eating and exercise and improves following rectal expulsion of gas and feces, rest, and application of heat to the abdomen. The second type of pain is colicky and is generally followed—and relieved—by a bowel movement or expulsion of gas. Pain is moderate in most cases, but its chronicity and persistence interfere with the quality of life and efficiency at work. At times some patients have such severe pain that it simulates an acute abdomen. The pain rarely occurs at night, nor does it awaken the patient. It begins in the early morning, when the colon ordinarily becomes active.

Meteorism is a common complaint. The patient refers to it as abdominal distention that makes it necessary to loosen or remove close-fitting garments. It begins in the morning and gradually increases as the day goes on, reaching its maximum in the evening. Passing gas, which is not always easy to do, relieves it temporarily. It usually occurs with constipation rather than with diarrhea and is made worse by the ingestion of greasy or highly spiced foods.

Constipation is rarely missing in patients with irritable bowel. Sometimes it alternates with diarrhea. It is characterized by small, dry stools. These findings, added to a feeling of incomplete defecation, impel patients to use laxatives excessively, thus complicating the clinical picture. Most of these medications are irritating and increase the pathophysiologic disturbances. As their action is temporary, the patient changes from one kind of laxative to another. The result is to aggravate the condition.

Diarrhea can alternate with constipation either spontaneously or from the effect of laxatives, or it may be the principal symptom. The desire to defecate is urgent and contrasts with the small volume of the stool. The feces are liquid or semisolid and contain varying amounts of mucus and undigested material. Evacuation is preceded by borborygmi and/or abdominal pain and may be followed by tenesmus. Most of the bowel movements occur in the early hours of the day and after eating (gastrocolic reflex). Nocturnal diarrhea does not occur.

Functional disturbances of the colon usually coincide with functional disturbances of other segments of the digestive tract and of other organs and systems that are under autonomic nervous control. Thus the patient may suffer gastric dyspepsia, functional disturbances of the small intestine, vascular disturbances, headaches, or neurodermatitis.

Functional disturbances of the colon do not affect the nutritional state. Patients look well even though the symptoms may have been present a long time. This finding clearly differentiates functional disturbances of the colon from inflammatory enteropathies and colopathies and from the malabsorption syndrome.

Studies by Almy et al 30 years ago showed clearly that colonic tone and motility are altered in patients with irritable colon. Constipation coincides with increased tone and is augmented by poorly synchronized contractions in the distal part of the colon, with resulting retention of feces. In cases of diarrhea, however, the propulsive action of the right colon is increased while the left distal segments are hypotonic with decreased motility, a combination that favors diarrhea. The pain is produced by distention or by spasm of the smooth muscles of the intestine.

Causes

Functional disturbances of the colon have many causes. Dietary indiscretions can upset the digestive system. An excess of irritating foods containing much undigestible matter, irregular hours of eating, and tachyphagia are said to be frequent causes. Not all believe this. Irritating foods containing much undigestible material appear to harm only those who are already suffering digestive disturbances from some other cause or who are not accustomed to that type of food. As to irregular hours and eating too fast, these may be signs of psychic tension and stress, which are often the primary cause of the functional disturbances. The same may be said about the abuse of laxatives. They merely aggravate a condition caused by other factors.

Secondary functional disturbances are those that follow some primary pathology. Nervous or humoral mechanisms may alter the function of the colon. Primary pathology in the internal female genitalia and urinary tract pathology in both sexes cause secondary functional disturbances of the colon. Hyperthyroidism, hypothyroidism, adrenal insufficiency, and hypercalcemia of any origin alter intestinal motility.

Iatrogenic causes are becoming more common in view of the increasing number of medications available. Medications altering intestinal physiology include anticholinergics, antihypertensives, antidepressives, codeine, thyroid hormones, antacids, and antibiotics, to name a few.

Although quite a few causes have been named, they are only a small fraction of the factors that may be involved in functional disturbances of the colon. Gastroenterologists agree that psychologic factors are the fundamental cause in the great majority of cases. The extraordinary frequency with which irritable colon coincides with other functional disturbances that characteristically fit into the picture of anxiety, depression, and obsessive-compulsive neurosis makes it quite probable that irritable colon is one of the clinical manifestations of neurosis.

If you evaluate the personality and character of patients suffering the irritable bowel syndrome and seek to discover emotional conflicts, you'll find frank evidence of neuroses in almost all of them. The majority have variable degrees of anxiety, and many others have depression, hypochondriasis, and obsessive-compulsive traits. From these observations it is not difficult to conclude that functional disturbances of the colon do not occur as isolated syndromes but as part of a larger picture. Often the diagnosis will vary with the type of specialist the patient consults. A gastroenterologist will diagnose irritable colon, a cardiologist will call it cardiac neurosis, and a psychiatrist will diagnose anxiety. On the other hand, very few individuals have not had functional disturbances of the colon. They occur in times of temporary stress, either external or internal. These short-term occasional, and unimportant, psychosomatic reactions obviously related to stress are not considered pathologic but merely as parts of a normal life.

Many theories have been advanced to explain why the colon is affected by stress. Individuals with irritable colon are thought to have a certain personality that was determined by a fixation at some stage of their psychosexual development. Fixation during the "anal stage," when the child is being toilet-trained, at times with accompanying severe punishment or exaggerated rewards, supposedly forms an "anal" personality. The "anal" personality is rigid, avaricious, obsessively neat and clean—and constipated. Other authors, basing their opinions on the study of many patients with irritable colon, have found that these patients are perfectionistic, hypersensitive, and excessively dependent on the opinion of others. When these individuals believe their ego is threatened or fear that their behavior will be criticized, they develop anxiety and guilt. In situations involving a real or imaginary injustice, they feel great resentment. Patients with irritable colon, then, are victims of anxiety, guilt feelings, and resentments.

On the other hand, it has been stated that no specific type of personality is related to irritable colon but that what is characteristic is the nature of the psychic conflict. Thus, those with constipation have conflicts that arouse hostility and resentment. Those with diarrhea react to conflict with guilt feelings and a tendency to weep and retreat from conflict. Other authors insist that the intestinal response is merely part of the total, integrated homeostatic defense reaction when the patient feels challenged by external or internal, real, anticipated, or imaginary threats. Finally, other investigators fail to find anything specific in either the personality or the psychic conflicts of these patients. The selection of the colon as the organ of expression of psychic stress is due to susceptibility because of "constitutional inferiority" or because some past organic illness has left it more vulnerable.

Abnormalities in basal electric rhythm have been demonstrated in the colonic musculature of patients with irritable colon. This suggests an intrinsic pathophysiologic abnormality that might precede and favor development of the clinical syndrome.

Diagnosis

The diagnosis of irritable colon should not be made lightly. Many sources of error exist. Similar symptoms are found in a large number of diseases both within the digestive tract and outside it. In addition, there are few examples in human pathology in which a complete diagnosis is more necessary to successful therapy. A complete diagnosis means that you cannot be content with giving the condition a name; it's necessary to understand the patient as a person and the stresses he is exposed to in order to ascertain the cause of the trouble. The following steps are recommended for arriving at a complete diagnosis:

1. Identification of the colon as the site where the symptoms originate
2. Thorough history and physical examination

3. Stool culture and at least three examinations for ova and cysts of parasites; in case of diarrhea, fresh stools should be examined for motile forms of *Entamoeba histolytica*
4. Proctosigmoidoscopy
5. Barium enema and small bowel series.

It is particularly important to rule out lactose intolerance and gluten enteropathy, which may be confused with irritable colon.

An attempt should be made to evaluate the patient from the psychological standpoint, to identify signs and symptoms of psychic tension and emotional conflict, to establish correlations between symptoms and emotional reactions, and to identify the conflicts at home, school, work, social life, and elsewhere. This list of data may seem too formidable and impractical, especially because of the limited time allotted to each patient and the scarcity of physicians with some psychiatric training. However, the study can be done gradually in the course of various examinations and interviews. Most patients are eager to be viewed as persons, rather than body systems, and want to develop such a relationship with their physician. They seek understanding and sympathy. Such communication is of great therapeutic value.

Treatment

Cardinal points in the traditional treatment of functional disorders of the colon are a bland diet, sedative and antispasmodic medication, and physical and mental rest. For constipation, mild laxatives of the mechanical type are prescribed, such as psyllium seeds and methylcellulose. Irritating laxatives are strictly forbidden. Correct habits of elimination are encouraged. For diarrhea, intestinal astringents and antidiarrheals are prescribed. Meals should be eaten at regular hours. Any dental problems should be attended to. Patients are usually told that they have no organic illness and that there is really nothing wrong with them. They are advised to stop fretting, avoid problems and difficulties, and try to enjoy themselves and take frequent vacations. Most of these recommendations prove to be effective. With this regimen, the symptoms may improve and even subside completely.

When functional digestive symptoms are part of the clinical syndrome of anxiety, depression, or any other psychologic disease, as is usually the case, these measures are not enough. The recommendation to enjoy life, rest, and, above all, avoid worry and problems is a bit naive. The statement that there is nothing organically wrong, that the problem is all mental, is perceived by such a patient as an insult or, at least, as a lack of understanding. The frustrated patient looks for another physician, at times engaging in an endless search for help. Study of the patient along the lines described in Chapter 12 is the basis for psychotherapy; this is the fundamental treatment in these cases. During these interviews the patient discovers for himself the relationship between his symptoms and his psychic tension and begins to understand the mechanism of his disease. Encouraged, he begins to talk about his conflicts and to recognize his fears and stresses, learning to communicate his emotions both verbally and nonverbally. A sympathetic atmosphere and the patient's acceptance of the doctor as a person who is interested in him and wants to understand him are of enormous therapeutic value. Often this is all the psychotherapy necessary to cure the patient.

In some patients, however, the conflicts are so serious and profound that they need specialized psychiatric help. Even so, a physician who recognizes the psychologic problems of his patients can teach them the true origin of their symptoms and guide them on the road to recovery.

The importance of the new psychotherapeutic agents should not be underestimated. Both the tranquilizers and the antidepressives, if carefully selected and used with skill, in combination with a psychotherapeutic attitude, are very effective in functional disturbances of the digestive tract.

Bibliography

Almy TP: Experimental studies on the irritable colon. *Am J Med* 10:60, 1951

Blackwell B: Psychosomatic aspects of gastrointestinal complaints. *J Ky Med Assoc* 74:26, 1976

Hislop IG: Psychological significance of the irritable colon syndrome. *Gut* 12:452, 1971

Palmer RI, Stonehill E, Cresp AH, et al: Psychological characteristics of patients with the irritable bowel syndrome. *Postgrad Med J* 50:416, 1974

Snape JW Jr, Carlson MG, Cohen S: Colonic myoelectric activity in the irritable bowel syndrome. *Gastroenterology* 70:326, 1976

White BP, Cobb S, Jones CM: Mucous colitis. *Psychosom Med Monogr* 1, 1939

SUMMARY

Functional, nonorganic disturbances of the colon, or "irritable colon," occur at any age, more frequently in women and young adults. After age 50, the diagnosis should be questioned. Various combinations of symptoms occur: abdominal pain, meteorism, constipation, diarrhea, small stools, sensation of incomplete evacuation, mucus in the stools. These may be continuous or intermittent with exacerbations and remissions for years. Usually functional difficulties of other parts of the gastrointestinal tract or other organs or systems are also present. These patients almost all show signs of neurosis. Nutritional state is almost never affected. Why the colon is selected as the site of the neurosis is still in question. This condition should be diagnosed only after very careful study since there are organic conditions that present a similar clinical picture. Supportive treatment and psychotherapy are in order.

Hyperthyroidism

57

Patients with hyperthyroidism often have a slight increase in the
number of bowel movements, which are of the usual consistency. This tendency corrects any constipation that may
have existed before the onset of the disease. A smaller sub-
group of hyperthyroid individuals exists in whom diarrhea
is the principal symptom while the other signs of hyperthyroidism are so mild that they may go unnoticed, making the
diagnosis difficult.

Hyperthyroid diarrhea is characterized by its chronicity
and resistance to symptomatic therapy. The patient loses
weight. If other, previously unnoticed signs of hyperthyroidism are looked for, they will be found: tachycardia, ex-

cess sweating, tremor, enlargement of the thyroid gland, and exophthalmos. Antithyroid therapy results in prompt subsidence of the diarrhea.

The cause of diarrhea in hyperthyroidism is unknown. A relationship between the exaggerated activity of the sympathetic nerves sometimes seen in this endocrine disease has been proposed. However, overactivity of the sympathetic nerves should inhibit rather than stimulate intestinal activity. The fact that the basic electrical rhythm in the intestine has an abnormal number of "slow waves" may be more significant. On the other hand, it should be remembered that recent studies of the pathophysiologic mechanisms of diarrhea have shown, in the majority of cases, that these are not motor problems but problems related to the transport of water and electrolytes across the intestinal membrane. This is the direction further investigation should take in solving the origin and pathogenesis of diarrhea in hyperthyroidism.

Bibliography

Christensen J, Schedl HP, Clifton JA: The basic electrical rhythm of the human duodenum in normal subjects and in patients with thyroid disease. *J Clin Invest* 43:1659, 1964

Diabetic diarrhea

58

The diabetic patient may suffer from many kinds of diarrheal syndromes (Table 58-1). A specific entity does, however, exist that deserves the name "diabetic diarrhea."

Two diarrheal syndromes related to diabetes are pancreatic diarrhea (Chapter 55) and celiac sprue (Chapter 40). When the mass of pancreatic tissue has been reduced by disease to the point where there is exocrine insufficiency, there may also be endocrine insufficiency. Diarrhea and steatorrhea, on the one hand, and diabetes, on the other, have a common etiology. Medical management endeavors to compensate for both deficiencies by supplying the enzymes and the hormone.

TABLE 58-1

Causes of diarrhea
and steatorrhea in diabetics

Recurring intestinal infections
Visceral neuropathy
Associated celiac sprue
Motility disturbances, with bacterial overgrowth
Exocrine pancreatic insufficiency
Vascular insufficiency of the intestine
Anal incontinence

Some studies show that the coincident occurrence of diabetes and celiac sprue is greater than would be expected from chance. No other information is available that suggests a possible relationship between the two. From a practical point of view, the problem consists of determining the cause of steatorrhea in diabetic patients. This should be solved by doing the indicated intestinal absorption tests, a peroral biopsy of the small intestinal mucosa, and therapeutic trials of pancreatic extract or a gluten-free diet.

Diabetic diarrhea usually has its onset in relatively young people, between the ages of 20 and 40, who have had longtime hyperglycemia that was difficult to control. They nearly always have retinopathy and nephropathy and always have diabetic neuropathy. This neuropathy involves not only the peripheral nerves but also the autonomic nervous system ("autonomic neuropathy"). The results are sensory and tendon reflex changes, sexual impotence, orthostatic hypotension, and disturbance of the pupillary reflexes and sphincters. Diarrhea is liquid, abundant, and predominantly nocturnal. It occurs with unpredictable exacerbations and remissions. It does not respond to antidiarrheal medication. Pancreatic extracts are of no value since it is not caused by exocrine pancreatic insufficiency. Gluten-free diets have no effect. Broad-spectrum antibiotics occasionally help, but only temporarily.

It is important to differentiate clearly between diabetic diarrhea and rectal incontinence caused by changes in the anal sphincter. This is a common complication of visceral neuropathy and when it is combined with diarrhea it presents an extremely difficult therapeutic problem.

Bibliography

Katz LA, Spiro HM: Gastrointestinal manifestations of diabetes. *N Engl J Med* 275:1350, 1966

McNally EF, Reinhard AE, Schwartz PE: Small bowel motility in diabetes. *Am J Dig Dis* 14:163, 1969

Whalen GE, Soergel KH, Geenen EJ: Diabetic diarrhea. A clinical and pathophysiological study. *Gastroenterology* 56:1021, 1969

SUMMARY

Diabetic diarrhea usually occurs in long-term diabetics between the ages of 20 and 40, in whom hyperglycemia has been difficult to control. There are concomitant retinopathy, nephropathy, and neuropathy. The diarrhea is liquid, voluminous, and mostly nocturnal. Celiac sprue is found more commonly among diabetics than in the general population, but no relationship has been proved.

PART IV

APPENDICES

Appendix A

Procto-sigmoidoscopic technique

Preparation

In patients with diarrhea, it is preferable to do the examination without preparatory laxatives or enemas. This gives a dependable picture of the rectal and sigmoid mucosa unaffected by the irritation of these procedures. The abundant liquid feces that may obstruct the view may be removed by aspiration or with cotton swabs. If no pathologic lesions are found and if the study is not satisfactory because of feces in the rectum and sigmoid, a simple saline enema or an enema of sodium phosphate, available commercially, is given to empty the rectum and sigmoid completely and make it possible to see any localized lesions, especially polyps and malignant growths, that otherwise would be missed.

Position of the patient

Three positions are recommended. The most comfortable for both patient and physician is to kneel on the proctology table.

Another excellent position is the knee-chest, which can be held on any examining table, even on a bed. The patient must rest on one shoulder, usually the left, the thighs must be vertical, the knees separated 10 to 15 cm. Some patients are so weak that they cannot maintain this position. In that case they can lie on the left side with the right knee and hip in complete flexion, the left knee and hip slightly flexed, and the gluteal area on a line with or projecting slightly beyond the border of the table or bed.

Instruments

The best instrument is, of course, the one the physician is accustomed to. Many prefer a sigmoidoscope 25 cm long and 2 cm in diameter with proximal illumination or fiberglass. In patients with stenotic lesions, smaller calibers such as the pediatric type should be used.

Technique

The rectum must be palpated before the instrument is introduced. This not only gives valuable information regarding the rectal walls but also relaxes the rectal sphincter and assures the examiner that there is no obstacle that would make introduction of the instrument dangerous. The instrument, well lubricated, is then introduced perpendicular to the anus with its point directed toward the umbilicus, and gentle, consistent pressure is applied. After the resistance of the anal sphincter is overcome, the instrument is pushed in a few centimeters and the obturator withdrawn. It is then introduced further, with its progress guided visually. All attention should be directed to the insertion of the instrument, and none to any pathology, which is observed as the instrument is withdrawn. The distal 15 cm corresponding to the rectum offers no resistance to the passage of the instrument, which has only to pass the borders of the valves of Houston. At the rectosigmoid junction, however, the intestine not only narrows but sometimes forms an angle so sharp that it is difficult to pass. Moderate insufflation of air can be of great help.

The rigid sigmoidoscope has several drawbacks: Its introduction is associated with unavoidable discomfort. On average, it reaches only 25 cm, frequently even less. This often is not far enough to see diverticular disease, strictures, localized inflammatory bowel disease, polyps, or colon cancer. The flexible fiberoptic pansigmoidoscope, on the other hand, may be inserted three times as far into the colon (60 cm). It is better tolerated than the rigid sigmoidoscope, and its diagnostic yield is far superior. It offers promise as a practical diagnostic tool in patients with suspected colorectal diseases.

Bibliography

Bohlman TW, Katon RM, Lipshutz GR, et al: Fiberoptic pansigmoidoscopy. An evaluation and comparison with rigid sigmoidoscopy. *Gastroenterology* 72:644, 1977

Winnan G, Berci G, Panish J, et al: Superiority of the flexible to the rigid sigmoidoscope in routine proctosigmoidoscopy. *N Engl J Med* 302:1011, 1980

Appendix B

Peroral biopsy of the small intestine

Preparation

The patient must be fasting. Bleeding tests must be normal. The patient should be told what to expect. This helps greatly to calm him and obtain his cooperation.

Instruments

Various types of instruments have been used. Of these, many prefer Carey's capsule and Quinton's instrument.

Carey's capsule

This instrument is 2.4 cm long by 0.8 cm in diameter. It is shaped like a medicinal capsule and its two halves, made of stainless steel, are held together by a spring (Figure B-1). It is closed by slipping one half over the other. The external half has an orifice, or window, into which a piece of intestinal mucosa is pulled if sufficient negative pressure is applied inside the capsule. The internal half has a sharp border that acts as a knife, cutting off the fragment of mucosa in

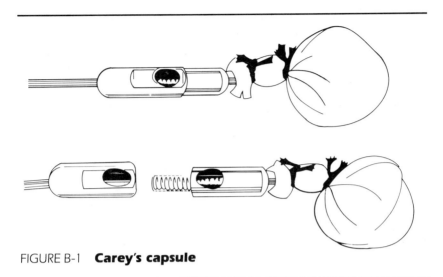

FIGURE B-1 **Carey's capsule**

the window when negative pressure moves the internal toward the external half. At its distal end, the capsule has a la-
tex bag containing mercury to facilitate its transit toward
the intestine. The proximal end is connected to a
polyethylene tube sufficiently long to permit the capsule to
reach the small intestine.

So that the capsule reaches the site chosen for the biopsy,
generally the duodenojejunal angle, the patient is given
some water and asked to swallow. Once the capsule is swallowed it is allowed to go down some 60 cm with the patient
sitting, which ensures its arrival at the gastric antrum. To
help the capsule pass through the pylorus, the patient lies
on his right side with the hips elevated 30°. In this position
the capsule and its tube travel around the greater curvature
and reach the pylorus. The tube is allowed to slip in 2 to 3 cm
every five to 10 minutes. The proximal end of the tube
should be attached to a receptacle where the digestive juices
can be collected. When these become tinged with bile, the
capsule has reached the duodenum. When the length has
reached 85 to 90 cm, the capsule has arrived at the angle of
Treitz. This can be checked by a plain film of the abdomen
and, in case of doubt, by injecting through the tube a small
amount of soluble radiopaque solution.

To obtain the biopsy specimen, the proximal end of the tube is connected to a 100-ml syringe containing 20 to 30 ml of water or saline solution, which is injected vigorously to flush the system. Then traction is applied by pulling back on the plunger to the 100-ml mark and maintaining negative pressure for a few minutes. The tube is then slowly withdrawn while suction is maintained. The sustained action first pulls a piece of the mucosa into the window of the capsule, serving to seal the capsule. This creates negative pressure, which brings the two halves of the capsule together so that the sample of mucosa is sliced off. The procedure may be repeated several times as the capsule is withdrawn, in order to obtain several samples. Care must be taken to withdraw the tube only a few centimeters at a time, then apply suction, and repeat the procedure a few minutes later. When the capsule finally appears, it is opened and the slice(s) of mucosa removed.

Quinton's capsule

This instrument is preferable to Carey's capsule when several samples are desired. Thanks to a special hydraulic addition, these can be obtained without withdrawing the instrument. The apparatus is 120 cm long and 4.7 mm in diameter and works by suction. It has a traction wire connected to a cylindrical knife that cuts the mucosa (Figure B-2). The tube is sufficiently flexible to be guided toward the desired spot in the intestine under fluoroscopy. Its passage through the pylorus may be accomplished by the same methods used with Carey's capsule. When it has reached the duodenum, with the patient supine, the instrument is pushed until its border is about to cross the vertebral column from the right to the left side. The patient is then turned onto his left side, enabling the tip of the tube to reach the angle of Treitz quite easily. The capsule is then opened, the manometric syringe adjusted, and a small amount of air injected to check that the system is open. Then negative pressure is applied according to tables that have been worked out for this procedure. Suction is maintained for four seconds, whereupon the knife is closed and the biopsy cut.

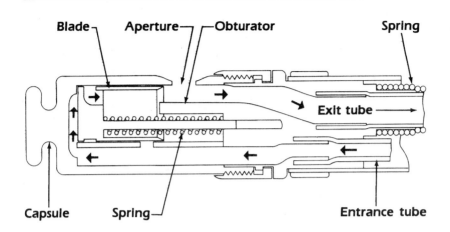

FIGURE B-2 **Schematic diagram of Quinton's biopsy capsule**
Negative pressure is applied through the exit tube so that the intestinal mucosa is sucked into the opening, is sectioned by the blade, and
is carried through the exit tube via a stream of water at a pressure that
penetrates the entrance tube and causes the blade to function. The
obturator limits the size of the mucosal fragments and reduces the risk
of perforation and hemorrhage

Care of the specimen

It's of prime importance to remove the specimen as soon as
possible, handling it with great care because of its extreme
fragility. Even more important is to place it on paper or
Gelfoam correctly, with the mucosal surface up. This en-
ables the pathologist to make perpendicular sections, which
are indispensable for correct histologic interpretation.
Oblique sections give a false image of shortened villi and
other artifacts and destroy the biopsy's value.

Complications

These are rare and consist of hemorrhage, bacteremia, and
perforation. Bleeding is generally moderate and is discovered only by testing for occult blood in the stool. Very rarely

is it macroscopic and severe. Bacteremia causes fever lasting a few hours. Perforation can be prevented if the window of the instrument is no larger than 2 mm in cases where the intestinal wall is suspected of being very thin, as in children and in advanced cases of celiac sprue with malnutrition.

Bibliography

Boyce HW, Palmer ED: *Techniques of Clinical Gastroenterology*, p 298. Springfield, Il: Thomas, 1975

Brandenborg LL, Rubin CE, Quinton WW: A multipurpose instrument for suction biopsy of the esophagus, stomach, small bowel and colon. *Gastroenterology* 37:1, 1959

Appendix C

Duodenal aspiration

A standard Rehfuss tube with an olive is used and is given to the patient to swallow until the first mark on the tube reaches his mouth, which indicates that the olive has reached his stomach. The gastric contents are then aspirated and the patient is asked to lie down on his right side and to push the tube in, at the rate of one inch every five minutes, until mark 3 reaches his lips. After a variable length of time, clear yellow fluid will flow from the tube. This indicates that the olive is in the right place. Then 30 ml of 33 per cent magnesium sulfate or olive oil are injected into the duodenum and the duodenal contents are allowed to drain out freely. Soon, dark bile appears. It is excellent material in which to look for parasites.

If it is difficult to place the olive in the duodenum, the following procedures are helpful: (1) elevating the patient's hips on a cushion or (2) placing the patient on his left side for 10 minutes and then on his right side. Following are two easy ways to locate the tip of the tube: (1) Have the patient take a few swallows of water. If this can be aspirated, the tube is in the stomach and should be withdrawn up to the first mark to begin again. (2) Connect a syringe to the tube and apply suction; if this creates a vacuum and no liquid is aspirated, it can be assumed that the olive is in the duodenum.

The ideal material for finding parasites is the mucus in the dark bile as well as in sedimented bile. The parasites most frequently found are *Giardia lamblia, Necator americanus, Ancylostoma duodenale,* and *Strongyloides stercoralis.*

Bibliography

Boyce HW, Palmer ED: *Techniques of Clinical Gastroenterology.* Springfield, Il: Thomas, 1975

Appendix D

Antidiarrheal medications

Since diarrhea is a symptom, all antidiarrheal drugs are merely symptomatic. Besides alleviating the symptom, they may prevent water and electrolyte imbalance. However, antidiarrheals are used too frequently instead of finding out the cause of the diarrhea and treating the underlying disease. It must be remembered that antidiarrheal drugs may be dangerous and even contraindicated. This is so in the acute bacterial diarrheas, where the infection becomes prolonged if it is artificially stopped, and in ulcerative colitis, where drastic antidiarrheal medicine can precipitate toxic megacolon. Antidiarrheal drugs, then, should not replace an adequate study of the patient nor should they be considered anything but a complement to treatment. They should be taken in moderation, with an understanding that the diarrhea is not the disease but one of its symptoms and, in many acute forms, a protective mechanism. Finally, be sure that the patient does not have a condition in which an antidiarrheal drug is contraindicated.

Common antidiarrheals

Kaolin and pectin

Although available separately, these are usually mixed in commercial antidiarrheal preparations (Kaopectate and others). Kaolin is a silicate of hydrated aluminum in native form. It is a white or yellow powdered clay and has been in use for more than 200 years as an adsorbent and protective. It has been claimed that kaolin adsorbs toxins, viruses, and bacteria, covers and protects the intestinal mucosa, and thickens the intestinal contents. No satisfactory scientific studies have been done to prove this. Clinical experience, however, does indicate that kaolin is a mild antidiarrheal that may be helpful.

Pectin is a carbohydrate obtained from a diluted acid extract of the inner layer of the rind of citrus fruits and from the residue of apple pulp. Chemically, it is made up of partially methoxylated polygalacturonic acids. Pectin dissolved in 20 parts of water forms a viscous acid colloid. The mechanism of its action is unknown. It is considered to be adsorptive and protective. Like kaolin, its value has not been scientifically proved; however, it is probably harmless.

Activated charcoal

This is the residue from destructive distillation of wood pulp. It has great adsorptive capacity because its particles are so small that it offers an enormous surface in proportion to its mass. This quality makes it a valuable antidote in poisoning. It adsorbs the poison quickly, before the gastrointestinal tract can do so. Here again, satisfactory scientific studies are lacking regarding its antidiarrheal value. It may contain impurities such as benzopyrene and methylcholanthrene, which are carcinogenic.

Attapulgite (Rheaban)

This is a silicate of aluminum and magnesium similar to kaolin and possesses the same pharmacologic properties. The dose is 6 to 9 gm/day.

Aluminum hydroxide

When aluminum hydroxide is used as an antacid, it causes constipation and so has been adopted as an antidiarrheal. Its effect is thought to be due to astringent qualities of aluminum salts. Astringents act locally, precipitating proteins, and so are said to reduce the permeability of the cellular membrane without damaging the cell. No proof exists that astringent properties are helpful in diarrhea or that aluminum hydroxide is an effective antidiarrheal.

Bismuth subnitrate and bismuth subsalicylate (Pepto-Bismol)

These salts are said to form a protective layer on the mucosa of the digestive tract, but this has not been proved either by animal studies or by human gastroscopy. As to their value as antidiarrheals, some uncontrolled studies seem to indicate that they are useful. In children, absorption of some of the nitrates of bismuth subnitrate can cause methemoglobinemia. Bismuth salts probably have mild antidiarrheal effects, but more complete studies should be done.

Calcium salts

A solution of calcium hydroxide known as lime water has been used as an antacid and is constipating. For this reason it has been used in the treatment of diarrhea. The same may be said of calcium carbonate.

Anticholinergics

Belladonna alkaloids, i.e., atropine, scopolamine, and *l*-hyoscyamine, their synthetic substitutes, and the quaternary ammonium compounds such as propantheline bromide (Pro-Banthine) are known to be constipating and have been used in the treatment of diarrhea. They are said to be especially useful against diarrhea caused by increased intestinal motility, as in irritable colon. However, even in this pathophysiologic disorder they are only mildly effective. Experiments on human subjects in whom intestinal motility was recorded showed that psychogenic stimuli caused motor disturbances that were not blocked by therapeutic doses of anticholinergics.

Opiates

Opium derivatives have been considered the antidiarrheals par excellence. It was thought that they slow intestinal transit by increasing nonpropulsive muscle activity. These drugs appear to cause increased rhythmic activity of intestinal circular muscles while perhaps inhibiting the contractility of longitudinal muscles. More recently the concept that the primary mechanism of the antidiarrheal action of opiates is on muscle has been seriously challenged. There is evidence that endogenous, natural, and synthetic opiates affect water and electrolyte transport by the intestine.

Opiates should be given only in diarrhea of short duration because of the risk of addiction. Most commonly used are several-times-daily doses of tincture of opium, 0.5 to 1 ml, or paregoric elixir, 5 to 10 ml. They may be dangerous in patients with ulcerative colitis because of the risk of producing toxic megacolon.

Diphenoxylate

This derivative of meperidine has antidiarrheal action intermediate between those of opiates and anticholinergics. It is available as Lomotil, containing 2.5 mg of diphenoxylate and 0.6 mg of atropine. The initial dose is two tablets four times a day. Diphenoxylate is less potent than codeine and more expensive. In acute diarrheas, it has no advantage over the opiates. In chronic diarrheas, however, it is superior because there is no danger of addiction.

Loperamide (Imodium)

Loperamide hydrochloride is a synthetic antidiarrheal that apparently acts by slowing intestinal motility. It inhibits peristaltic activity by a direct effect on the circular and longitudinal muscles of the intestinal wall. For acute diarrhea the recommended initial dose is 4 mg, followed by 2 mg after each unformed stool.

Frontiers in the pharmacologic treatment of diarrhea

The discovery that, contrary to previous belief, most diarrheal syndromes are due not to disturbances in intestinal motility but to abnormalities in fluid and electrolyte transport has led to an intensive search for pharmacologic agents that could reverse such pathophysiologic changes. A list of the more promising agents includes aspirin, indomethacin (Indocin), bismuth subsalicylate, nicotinic acid, chlorpromazine (Thorazine), and lithium carbonate. The therapeutic role of these agents, many of which have antiprostaglandin effects, remains to be established. There is no doubt, however, that a new frontier has been opened.

Bibliography

DuPont HL, Hornick RB: Adverse effect of Lomotil therapy in shigellosis. *JAMA* 226:1525, 1973

DuPont HL, Sullivan P, Pickering LK, et al: Symptomatic treatment of diarrhea with bismuth subsalicylate among students attending a Mexican university. *Gastroenterology* 73:715, 1977

Holmgren J, Lange S, Lonroth I: Reversal of cyclic AMP-mediated intestinal secretion in mice by chlorpromazine. *Gastroenterology* 75:1103, 1978

Jacoby HI, Marshal CH: Antagonism of cholera enterotoxin by antiinflammatory agents in the rat. *Nature* 235:163, 1972

Jaffe BM, Kopen DF, DeSchryver-Kecskemeti K, et al: Indomethacin-responsive pancreatic cholera. *N Engl J Med* 297:817, 1977

Pandol SJ, Korman LY, McCarthy DM, et al: Beneficial effect of oral lithium carbonate in the treatment of pancreatic cholera syndrome. *N Engl J Med* 302:1403, 1980

Portnoy BL, DuPont H, Pruitt D, et al: Antidiarrheal agents in the treatment of acute diarrhea in children. *JAMA* 236:844, 1976

Powell DW: Muscle or mucosa: The site of action of antidiarrheal opiates? *Gastroenterology* 80:406, 1981

Read AE: Antidiarrheal agents. *Practitioner* 206:67, 1971

Appendix E

Gluten-free diet

The objective is to eliminate completely the gluten of wheat, rye, and barley in the diets of patients with celiac sprue and other gluten intolerance states.

Foods that should be included in the daily diet

Meat, fruits, vegetables, eggs, potatoes, butter, permitted cereals, and milk and milk products—unless the patient has lactase deficiency—are necessary for good nutrition.

Foods that are permitted

Beverages. Coffee, tea, cocoa, carbonated beverages.

Bread. Bread and muffins made with corn, rice, potato, arrowroot, or soybean flour.

Cereals. Cereals made from rice, corn, hominy, soybean, or tapioca.

Desserts. Gelatin, fruit ices, homemade ice cream, custards, rice pudding, corn pudding, tapioca pudding, and crackers or cookies made without wheat, rye, or (in most cases) oat flour.

Fats. Butter, margarine, corn oil, olive and other vegetable oils, homemade mayonnaise, shortening.

Fruits. Any.

Meats, eggs, or cheese. Any (see "Foods that must be excluded").

Soups. Broth or bouillon, vegetable and cream soups thickened with cornstarch, arrowroot, or potato flour.

Sweets. Any except those prepared with excluded grain products.

Vegetables. Any.

Miscellaneous. Spices, garlic, dry mustard, salt, lemon, olives, nuts, sour pickles, popcorn, sugar, syrups, honey, jellies, preserves, candies, alcoholic drinks, peanut butter.

Foods that must be excluded

Beverages. Cereal beverages, cocoa mixes, malted milks, drinks made with malt, ale, or beer.

Flours. All flours made from wheat, rye, or barley.

Cereals, breads, cookies, crackers, pancakes, waffles, and pastries. All those that contain wheat, barley, or rye.

Desserts. Doughnuts, commercial ice cream, pies, puddings.

Meats. Meats, poultry, fish, or seafoods that are breaded or made into croquettes; sausages, cold meats, frankfurters; gravy thickened with flour.

Others. Cream soups unless they are made at home, canned soups, salad dressings thickened with wheat flour.

Gluten-free commercial products

The following list excludes those products containing wheat, rye, oats, and barley, as well as malt flavoring or extract. This list does not include all permissible commercial products; many more could be added. Nor are all the products listed below necessarily available in all parts of the United States. It's wise for patients to check labels for ingredients when purchasing packaged or canned products, since ingredients may change from time to time.

Beverages

Maxwell House, Yuban, Sanka, and Brim regular and instant coffee.
Start and Tang instant breakfast drink.
Twist imitation lemonade and orangeade mixes.
Kool-Aid soft drink mixes (regular and presweetened).

Meat, poultry, and fish dinners

Beechnut
Turkey rice dinner
Egg yolks with bacon
Split peas & ham dinner

Campbell's
Franks & beans
Old fashioned beans
Pork & beans

Gerber's
Turkey rice dinner
Vegetables & bacon
Vegetables & liver with bacon
Vegetables & turkey
Split peas with bacon
Vegetables & chicken
Vegetables and beef
Creamed cottage cheese with pineapple.

Heinz
Cottage cheese with
banana
Vegetables & bacon
Vegetables & ham
Vegetables & lamb
Split peas, vegetables &
bacon.

Swanson's
Boned chicken
Chunk white chicken
Chicken spread
Boned turkey
Chunks o' turkey.

Breads, cereals, and crackers

Beechnut
Rice cereal.

Gerber's
Rice cereal
Rice cereal with
applesauce and banana.

Kellogg's
Sugar corn pops.

Quaker
Puffed rice.

Soups

Campbell's
Bean with bacon
Beef broth
Black bean
Chicken with rice
Chicken gumbo
Consommé (beef)
Onion
Vegetable bean
Vegetable beef
Frozen fish chowder
Frozen oyster stew
Frozen old fashioned
vegetable with beef
Frozen green pea with ham.

Red Kettle
Potato Soup Mix
Onion Soup Mix.

Swanson's
Clear chicken broth.

Heinz
Chicken soup.

Ice cream

Sealtest
McDonald's

Howard Johnson's
Brock-Hall.

Desserts

Gerber's
Cherry vanilla pudding
Chocolate flavored
custard pudding
Dutch apple dessert
Orange pudding
Vanilla custard pudding.

Heinz
Tutti frutti
Custard pudding
Fruit dessert
Orange pudding
Pineapple orange
dessert.

Beechnut
Chocolate custard
dessert
Cottage cheese with
pineapple
Fruit dessert
Orange pineapple dessert
Pineapple desserts
Tropical fruit dessert
Natural fruit gels
Vanilla custard pudding.

General Foods
Instant puddings
Pudding and pie fillings
Tapioca puddings
Whip 'n Chill dessert
mixes
Jell-O
Gelatin salad mixes
D-zerta dietary
puddings, pie fillings,
and gelatin desserts.

Salad dressings

Hellmann's
Tartar sauce
French dressings
Cheddar-bleu cheese
dressing
Italian
Real mayonnaise.

Kraft's
Miracle Whip
French dressing
Roquefort.

General Foods
Good Seasons salad
dressing mixes
Open Pit barbeque
sauces.

Flours

Cellu
Rice flour
Wheat starch
Corn

Soybean flour
Tapioca
Potato starch.

Candy

Hershey's
Milk chocolate with
almonds
Semisweet chocolate.

Nestlés
Crunch milk chocolate.

DeMet's
Turtles.

Hollywood's
Butter Nut.

Kraft
Caramels.

Pearson's
Mint patty.

Brach
Chocolate mint.

Schutter's
Bit o' Honey.

Clark
Milk Duds.

Necco
Canada Mints.

Nabisco
Junior Mints.

Heide
JujyFruits.

Others
Chuckles
Tootsie Roll
Heath bar
Life Savers
Reeds (all flavors).

Miscellaneous

Minute Rice
Karo syrups
French's prepared
mustard
Hershey chocolate and
cocoa
Nestlé's chocolate and
cocoa

Betty Crocker au gratin
potatoes, Potato Buds,
scalloped potatoes,
Bugles, coconut pecan
frosting mix
Minute tapioca
Heinz catsup
Frito's corn chips
Baker's chocolate and
cocoa.

Appendix F

Total parenteral nutrition

History

There is a group of diseases of the digestive tract, many of them with diarrhea and malabsorption as the outstanding pathophysiologic symptoms, in which the life of the patient literally depends on parenteral feeding. In 1656 Sir Christopher Wren invented the intravenous technique by connecting a pig's bladder to the quill of a goose and injecting wine, beer, and solutions of opium intravenously into dogs. Two centuries elapsed before Claude Bernard took the next step and injected glucose solutions into animals. Fifty years passed before Biedl and Kraus, in 1896, injected the same solutions into man. More than 60 years ago the use of hydrolyzed protein products for intravenous feedings was proposed, but it took another quarter of a century to put it into practice. It was readily observed that intravenous mixtures of glucose and amino acids (obtained by protein hydrolysis) restored depleted plasma proteins, which could not be done with glucose solutions alone. These mixtures, however, were not sufficient to supply energy requirements, especially in patients subjected to stress, and to furnish amino acids to rebuild proteins. From 5 to 10 liters a day of these solutions would be required to take care of their needs—and that would overload the circulatory system. More concentrated solutions could not be used because they would seriously damage the endothelium of the peripheral veins.

Dudrick et al solved the problem and devised a practical method of total parenteral feeding by infusing concentrated solutions of scientifically balanced nutrients directly into the superior vena cava. In this way the normal balance could be maintained and growth and development assured without upsetting the fluid balance or causing phlebitis. This has been one of the most outstanding advances in modern therapy. Its importance in patients with digestive diseases cannot be overestimated.

Basic concepts

Normal adults need 35 calories and 0.8 gm of protein per kilogram of weight per day. A 70-kg man needs 2,500 calories and 56 gm of protein a day. The minimum protein requirement is only 0.4 gm/kg/day. Many modern hospitals prepare their own solutions. These hospitals and the commercial laboratories have replaced hydrolyzed proteins with synthetic amino acids, which are more easily absorbed than peptides and can be made up in more physiologic proportions. The commercial preparation Freamine contains 39 gm of protein and 227 gm of glucose per liter. One liter is given the patient the first day, 2 liters the second day, and, from then on, 3 liters/day. Solutions prepared in hospitals contain 50 per cent dextrose, 8 to 10 per cent amino acids, sodium, potassium, calcium, phosphorus, magnesium, and vitamins. Table F-1 gives the contents of such a solution. In addition, patients on total parenteral nutrition receive iron and vitamin K, intramuscularly.

Technique

The catheter is introduced into the right subclavian vein under the clavicle, and passed into the superior vena cava just

TABLE F-1

Model solution for total parenteral nutrition

Volume	1,000 ml
Energy	~1,000 kcal
Components:	
Glucose	200 gm
Protein hydrolysate (amino acids)	37.5 gm
Sodium (chloride or lactate)	40–50 mEq
Potassium (dihydrogen phosphate)	30–40 mEq
Calcium (gluconate)	4.5–9 mEq
Magnesium (sulfate)	4–8 mEq
Vitamins and minerals (added once a day)	
Vitamin A	5,000–10,000 IU
Vitamin D	400 IU
Vitamin E	10–15 IU
Vitamin K_1 (optional)	1–2 mg
Vitamin C	250–500 mg
Thiamine	25–50 mg
Niacin	50–100 mg
Riboflavin	5–10 mg
Pantothenic acid	12.5–25 mg
Pyridoxine	7.5–15 mg
Folic acid (optional)	0.5–1.5 mg
Vitamin B_{12} (optional)	0.01–0.03 mg
Iron (optional)	2–3 mg

---

above the auricle. It is checked by a chest X-ray. Strict aseptic technique must be followed during both insertion and maintenance of the catheter and site. A Micropore filter removes micropeptides and other undesirable particles. A carefully regulated pump controls the rate of infusion. The catheter should never be used for anything but parenteral feeding. Other solutions, transfusions, and medication should be given via other veins. The dressing should be changed every two to seven days, and the tubing every day. Absolutely nothing should disturb the catheter in the superior vena cava.

TABLE F-2

Indications for total parenteral nutrition

Diseases of the digestive system	Hypermetabolic states
Fistulae	Burns
Prolonged pancreatitis	Sepsis
Short bowel syndrome	Injuries
Inflammatory bowel disease	Neoplastic diseases
Prolonged postoperative paralytic ileus	Anorexia nervosa
Developmental defects or trauma	
of the digestive tract	
Prolonged infant diarrhea	

Each hospital should have a team in charge of parenteral nutrition. An internist, trained in nutrition, should be in charge. A surgeon should be responsible for inserting the catheter in the superior vena cava. The team should include a pharmacist who is in charge of preparing the solutions under strict aseptic technique, preferably under a laminar flow hood, and a nurse who is responsible for meticulous care of the catheter. There must be a procedure manual that meets accreditation requirements.

The patient must be closely observed and careful records should be kept in regard to:

☐ Daily weight, vital signs, intake and output, urine glucose and acetone

☐ Twice weekly serum glucose, sodium, potassium, chloride, bicarbonate, calcium, and phosphorus

☐ Weekly blood count, plus serum creatinine and magnesium.

Indications for total parenteral nutrition

Indications are listed in Table F-2. Digestive diseases with diarrhea or malabsorption occupy an important place in the list. Total parenteral nutrition is essential during the adaptive stage in patients with short bowel (Chapter 44) and may be of outstanding value in the inflammatory enteropathies and colopathies, allowing patients to gain strength in preparation for surgery, to maintain their nutritional balance during acute exacerbations, or possibly to give the intestine a complete rest in order to hasten healing.

Complications

Complications may be classified as local, infectious, and metabolic. Local complications have to do with improper placing of the catheter, which may cause pneumothorax, hemothorax, hydrothorax, arteriovenous fistulae, damage to the brachial plexus, gas emboli, or emboli from fragments of the catheter. Thrombosis and phlebitis are two other possibilities.

Most patients requiring parenteral alimentation are in poor condition, being malnourished and having received antibiotics, corticosteroids, chemotherapeutic agents, and/or radiation therapy. This makes them easy prey to infection. Furthermore, with an indwelling catheter and intravenous solutions—especially the rich hyperalimentation solution— there is always the danger of introducing pathogenic organisms. A clinical rule should be that the sudden appearance of fever in a patient on total parenteral nutrition is due to the catheter until proved otherwise. The following steps should be taken:

1. The bottle containing the hyperalimentation solution should be replaced by glucose solution and the hyperalimentation bottle and tubing should be sent to the laboratory for culture
2. Blood should be drawn for cultures
3. Other causes of fever should be investigated
4. If the fever continues and no cause is found, blood should be taken directly from the catheter and cultured
5. The catheter should be withdrawn and a culture taken from its tip. If the fever subsides soon afterward, the catheter was probably contaminated with bacteria or fungi.

TABLE F-3

Metabolic complications
of total parenteral nutrition

Glucose
  Hyperosmolar coma
  Hypoglycemia
Amino acids
  Hyperammonemia
  Hyperazotemia
  Hyperchloremic acidosis
Essential fatty acids
  Deficiency

Calcium and phosphorus
  Hypercalcemia
  Hypophosphatemia
Hepatic steatosis
Trace elements
  Copper and zinc deficiencies
Vitamins
  Vitamin A and D intoxication

Metabolic complications are listed in Table F-3. If a hypertonic solution of glucose and amino acids is given too fast or if the patient's capacity to metabolize glucose is decreased, he may develop hyperglycemia with consequent osmotic glycosuria and diuresis and a hyperosmolar coma. For that reason it is very important to test regularly for glycosuria and glycemia. Supplemental insulin is sometimes given if the patient cannot metabolize the excess glucose. Large amounts of concentrated glucose given intravenously also stimulate the secretion of insulin. If the infusion is suddenly stopped, it could cause dangerous hypoglycemic shock. This is why total parenteral feedings must be begun and discontinued gradually.

A patient with impaired liver function may develop hyperammonemia. Hyperchloremic acidosis has been seen in young children when metabolism of the amino acids in the solution liberates excessive amounts of hydrogen ions. Excessive amounts of calcium or vitamin D cause hypercalcemia, a metabolic disturbance that can result in acute pancreatitis or hypercalciuria and kidney stones. Furthermore, if a patient with advanced malnutrition receives glucose and amino acids without sufficient phosphorus, he will consume his extracellular phosphorus stores with resulting hypophosphatemia and consequent paresthesias, weakness, confusion, convulsions, and even death.

When parenteral feeding is prolonged, a deficiency of essential fatty acids may occur. The skin becomes scaly and eczematous and the patient develops anemia and thrombocytopenia. These symptoms respond promptly to correction of the deficiency with linoleic acid by mouth or by applying sunflower oil to the skin since it is rich in that fatty acid. Another way of curing a deficiency of essential fatty acids is to give lipids intravenously. This is necessary in patients who are on total parenteral nutrition and have hepatomegaly and increases in transaminases and alkaline phosphatase. Liver biopsies from these patients show fatty infiltration, which has been attributed to excessive mobilization of fatty acids coming from fatty tissue to the liver, to increased synthesis of lipids in this organ, or to their decreased oxidation. Cases of copper deficiency and possibly zinc deficiency reveal our ignorance as to the basic requirements for these metals.

Partial parenteral nutrition

Solutions of electrolytes and 5 per cent glucose have the great advantage of being harmless to peripheral veins but they cannot maintain adequate nutrition. The solutions used for total parenteral feeding have solved the problem of nutrition but their high osmolarity (1,800 mOsM) makes it impossible to give them via peripheral veins. They must be given via the superior vena cava, a route not without complications. Fortunately, many patients can be fed partially by vein and partially by mouth, which makes the problem of maintaining nutrition easier to solve.

An intermediate method combining the advantages but not the disadvantages of both procedures has been devised and is of much value to patients with digestive disturbances. The solution is made up of glucose, amino acids, and minerals. It has an osmolarity of 900 mOsM, from which it takes the name P-900. Table F-4 compares P-900 with the conventional 5 per cent dextrose in saline.

TABLE F-4

Comparative compositions of solution P-900 and 5 per cent glucose in saline

Solution	Osmolarity (mOsM)	Electrolytes (mEq/liter)					P (gm/liter)	Glucose (gm/liter)	Amino acid N (gm/liter)
		Na	Cl	K	Mg	Ca			
P-900	900	50	45	40	8	7	200	65	4.13
Glucose in saline	400	35	55	20	0	0	0	50	0

The osmolarity of P-900 is moderately irritating to the venous epithelium. The addition of hydrocortisone, 5 mg/liter, decreases the venous inflammatory response so that the solution can be tolerated. Of course, P-900 does not have the same nutritional or caloric value as total hyperalimentation solutions and cannot be used as the only source of nutrition. It is therefore used as a supplement for patients who are able to take some food by mouth.

Ambulatory or home parenteral nutrition

Ambulatory or home parenteral nutrition has permitted the rehabilitation of patients with extensive intestinal resection, multiple fistulae, Crohn's disease, and scleroderma. While short-term total parenteral nutrition has been used widely in hospitalized patients for over a decade, home parenteral nutrition had to wait for the development of techniques allowing prolonged access to the central venous system. After implantation of a Silastic catheter, the patient and those responsible for home care must be taught proper aseptic technique in handling the catheter, sterile solutions, and the infusion system. Infusion may be regulated by either a pump, gravity drip, or pneumatic cuff device. The usual regimen consists of infusion of 2 to 3 liters of a sterile nutrient solution over 10 to 12 hours each night.

Bibliography

Broviac JW, Scribner BH: Prolonged parenteral nutrition in the home. *Surg Gynecol Obstet* 139:24, 1974

Dudrick SJ, Ruberg RL: Principles and practices of parenteral nutrition. *Gastroenterology* 61:901, 1971

Dudrick SJ, Wilmore DW, Vars HM, et al: Long-term total parenteral nutrition with growth, development and positive nitrogen balance. *Surgery* 64:134, 1968

Fleming RC, Beart RW Jr, Berkner S, et al: Home parenteral nutrition for management of the severely malnourished adult patient. *Gastroenterology* 79:11, 1980

Fleming RC, McGill DB, Hoffman HN, et al: Total parenteral nutrition. *Mayo Clin Proc* 51:187, 1976

Jeejeebhoy KN, Langer B, Tsallas G, et al: Total parenteral nutrition at home: Studies in patients surviving 4 months to 5 years. *Gastroenterology* 71:943, 1976

Solassol CL, Joyeux H, Etco L, et al: New techniques for long-term intravenous feeding: An artificial gut in 75 patients. *Ann Surg* 179:519, 1974

Index

Other titles of related interest from MEDICAL ECONOMICS BOOKS

Physicians' Guide to Diseases of the Oral Cavity— Illustrated
Harriet S. Goldman, D.D.S., M.P.H., and
Michael Z. Marder, D.D.S.
ISBN 0-87489-240-6

Physicians' Guide to Oculosystemic Diseases: Ophthalmoscopic Physical Diagnosis
William V. Delaney Jr., M.D.
ISBN 0-87489-250-3

Foreign Travel & Immunization Guide, 11th Edition
Hans H. Neumann, M.D.
ISBN 0-87489-262-7

Prescriber's Handbook of Therapeutic Drugs
Harry Swartz, M.D.
ISBN 0-87489-190-6

Outline Guide to Antimicrobial Therapy
John E. McGowan Jr., M.D.
ISBN 0-87489-249-X

Emotional Disorders: An Outline Guide to Diagnosis and Pharmacological Treatment
Alberto DiMascio, Ph.D., and Harold Goldberg, M.D.
ISBN 0-87489-147-7

Core Pathology: Fundamental Concepts and Principles
Chandler Smith, M.D.
ISBN 0-87489-239-2

Human Disease in Color
Chandler Smith, M.D.
ISBN 0-87489-188-4

For information, write to:

Medical Economics Books
680 Kinderkamack Road
Oradell, New Jersey 07649